The International Library of Psychology

A SHORT HISTORY OF
PSYCHOTHERAPY

T0221291

Founded by C. K. Ogden

The International Library of Psychology

ABNORMAL AND CLINICAL PSYCHOLOGY
In 19 Volumes

A SHORT HISTORY OF PSYCHOTHERAPY

In Theory and Practice

NIGEL WALKER

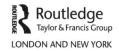

Routledge
Taylor & Francis Group

LONDON AND NEW YORK

First published in 1957
by Routledge

Reprinted in 1999
by Routledge
2 Park Square, Milton Park, Abingdon, Oxon, OX14 4RN

Simultaneously published in the USA and Canada by Routledge

711 Third Avenue, New York, NY 10017

Transferred to Digital Printing 2005

First issued in paperback 2013

The publishers have made every effort to contact authors/copyright holders
of the works reprinted in the *International Library of Psychology*.
This has not been possible in every case, however, and we would
welcome correspondence from those individuals/companies
we have been unable to trace.

These reprints are taken from original copies of each book. In many cases
the condition of these originals is not perfect. The publisher has gone to
great lengths to ensure the quality of these reprints, but wishes to point
out that certain characteristics of the original copies will, of necessity, be
apparent in reprints thereof.

British Library Cataloguing in Publication Data
A CIP catalogue record for this book
is available from the British Library

A Short History of Psychotherapy

ISBN 978-0-415-20936-6 (hbk)
ISBN 978-0-415-85065-0 (pbk)

TO

MY WIFE

CONTENTS

LIST OF PLATES

PREFACE

I T may reduce the number of disappointed readers if I use this preface to say what this book is not. For example, it is not a history of the kind which contains the names, biographical details and major publications of every psychotherapist from Mesmer to Rogers; these are included only where they seem to have a genuine bearing on the development of psychotherapy. Nor is it a pre-history; I do not really believe that the priests of Egypt or Epidaurus have had any important influence on twentieth-century theory or technique. Still less is it a manual of instruction for those who have decided on psychotherapy as a profession or a means of salvation; at most, it may help psychotherapists to be more flexible in their choice of method, and patients to be less discouraged if they fail to benefit from the technique of one particular school. Finally, it is not an account of all the psychological and philosophical theories of the psychotherapists. Since psychotherapy is a technique and not a science, I have aimed at tracing the development of the technical differences between the schools, and have dealt only with such theoretical disagreements as seemed to me to be connected with these technical differences. If anything, this has increased rather than lessened my difficulties. The literature of psychotherapy is profuse on the subject of theory and scanty on technique, so that in order to discover what this or that practitioner really does with his patients it is usually necessary to study a large number of theoretical essays, and even then to do a good deal of reading between the lines.

This may explain and justify some of the peculiarities of this book and, in particular, the omission of one or two well-known names and the inclusion of some less familiar ones. The men who were responsible for genuine innovations in technique are fewer than appears from the bibliographies, and are not always those who figure most frequently in them. Moreover, the space I have devoted to each school and each innovator is not necessarily proportionate to their importance at the present time (which may after all be out-of-date before long). If a technique seems to be logically distinct from the others I have given it enough space to make its distinctive features clear, even if it is represented today by no more than a handful of inbred survivors.

I have explained in their historical context the chief technical terms used by the schools of psychotherapy. Because there has so far been very little comparative study of these schools I have had to coin a few technical terms of my own, but I have kept them to a minimum and explained them. Any other psychiatric or psychological terms will be found in the Penguin *Dictionary of Psychology*.

Apart from the documentary sources which I have acknowledged in their place, I owe a great deal to the personal assistance which I have received from a large number of people. My particular thanks are due to:

Mr. Maurice Ash for information about the Withymead Centre; Dr. Jean Biggar of Edinburgh for reading the chapter on Group Psychotherapy and the appendix on Child Psychotherapy; Miss M. Cookson of Edinburgh University for references; Professor Rudolf Dreikurs of Chicago Medical School for information about Individual Psychology and Group Psychotherapy; Dr. Michael Fordham for criticisms of the chapters on Analytical Psychology; Dr. W. R. D. Fairbairn of Edinburgh for criticisms of the chapter on Post-Freudian Psychoanalysis; Dr. H. Guntrip of Leeds for criticisms of the chapters on Psychoanalysis; Mr. Hans Illing of Los Angeles for information about Group Psychotherapy; Professor Alexander Kennedy of Edinburgh University for information about Individual Psychology in Britain; Mrs. Melanie Klein for information about the development of her methods; Miss M. de Lepervanche, Library Secretary at the Institute of Psychoanalysis in London, for references; Miss A. M. Weil of the Hampstead Clinic, London, for references; Dr. F. N. L. Poynter of the Wellcome Historical Medical Library in London for references; Miss J. Hardman for typing the final text and correcting many mistakes.

Perhaps the best way in which I can repay their help is by making it clear that they are not responsible for the use which I have made of it.

December, 1956

I

INTRODUCTION

PSYCHIATRY, PSYCHOTHERAPY AND PSYCHOLOGY

THIS is a history of one particular sub-division of remedial medicine. Throughout the period of its development medicine has divided disorders into two main categories—those for which it could offer a physical cause (such as a broken bone or an infected liver) and those for which it could not. In the nineteenth century, when scientific advances were rapidly discovering physical causes for many hitherto unexplained phenomena, orthodox European physicians tended to consider that a disorder with no discoverable bodily cause was simply one about which we did not know enough, and wherever possible they tried to supply a bodily cause, often on very slender evidence. When they could not do this, the disorder was left to be treated by quacks or psychiatrists, who were not as clearly distinguished as they are today. These disorders included the delusions, irrational behaviour or unaccountable misery of the maniac, and the faintings, paralyses, convulsions and other physical symptoms of the hysteric or neurasthenic—all of them disorders which neither reasoning nor physical treatment could cure. The psychiatrists experimented with measures aimed at the patient's body—rest, light work, good food, massage or electric stimulation of the muscles; and when they had a certain amount of success with a particular disorder they felt that they had brought it within the respectable ambit of medicine. Meanwhile a few of the quacks were experimenting with a method that consisted of talking to the patient. They began by treating the more physical symptoms, but gradually extended forms of the technique to certain disorders of emotion, perception and behaviour. Eventually the technique was accepted by the orthodox psychiatrists as a way of treating the decreasing but more and more intractable residuum of disorders for which no really effective or permanent physical cure had been discovered. It is with the development of this semantic technique, which communicates with the patient instead of treating his body, that this book is concerned.

The modern descendants of the physical methods I have mentioned consist, broadly speaking, of treatment by drugs (for example, the induction of coma by insulin); by electrical stimulation of the brain (electro-convulsion); by surgery (for example, the partial severance of the frontal lobes from the rest of the brain); or by rest and segregation.. There is no universally accepted term for all these methods, and perhaps it will be safest and most precise if I simply refer to them as 'non-semantic treatment'. Together with the semantic methods they make up what is called 'psychiatry'. The semantic methods are usually grouped together under the heading of 'psychotherapy', and its different variations have names conferred by their inventors. Freud's name for his was 'psychoanalysis'; Adler's 'individual psychology'; Jung's 'analytical psychology'; Roger's 'non-directive therapy'. The use of the term 'psychology', however, for a remedial method is becoming increasingly unfashionable, and precise modern usage reserves it for the scientific study of human and animal behaviour.[1]

TECHNIQUES AND SCIENCES

This last distinction—between psychology and psychiatry—is an extremely important one for a proper understanding of the rest of this book. Psychology is a science and psychiatry is not. I do not mean that psychiatry is something which, if it makes good progress and does not misbehave, will one day be worthy of the name of science; for it is something quite different. It is a technique. The difference between sciences and techniques is not fully appreciated by many people who practise or talk about either, and this has given rise to quite a few misunderstandings, particularly in the field of medicine and psychotherapy. In order to make sense of the history of psychotherapy it is essential to be clear about the distinction, and as it has not been properly discussed in any book that I have read, I shall have to discuss it in this one.

[1] Or, to be more precise still, such aspects of it as are not studied by anthropologists, economists, ethologists and so forth.

A technique is a collection of rules for achieving a certain class of objectives. Strategy is the technique of winning wars; when we talk of 'our strategy' in the last war we mean the way in which we applied this technique to its particular circumstances. Carpentry is the technique of making or repairing things of wood. Each of these techniques is a system of rules which describe the means to those particular ends. In contrast, a science consists of a system of statements which either describe or explain observed phenomena. The science of genetics describes and explains the phenomena of the inheritance of characteristics in the propagation of living organisms. Sciences are defined by reference to their subject-matter, techniques by reference to their ends.

The distinction between a science and a technique has been obscured by people who have treated sciences as if they were glorified techniques—who would, for example, define genetics as the technique of breeding plants and animals so as to accentuate desirable characteristics and eliminate undesirable ones.[1] It is quite true that most of the sciences grew up as the result of a need to achieve some end or other. The very name of geometry, for example, betrays its humble origin in the need to have a technique for determining the areas of plots of land.[2] It is also true that a good deal of scientific research is carried on for highly practical reasons; nuclear physics is an obvious example. Again, almost all sciences make use of techniques in their experiments; genetics, for example, involves the very practical technique of keeping the experimental animals in good condition. Some techniques, too, are very 'scientific' in the way in which their rules are formulated; the technique of making optical instruments, such as microscopes, involves a lot of complicated rules about the curvature and position of lenses, as well as their chemical composition. But the distinction becomes clear again if we consider the relationship between any technique and any science with which it is connected. No technique is indissolubly linked to any one science. Even the nineteenth-century technique of making microscopes involved both the science of geometrical optics, with its focal lengths and

---

[1] Confusion has also been caused by the use of the term 'applied science' to include techniques. In its proper usage, an 'applied science' is a selection of the statements of a science which are likely to be of use to a particular technique or group of techniques.

[2] I realize that there is a logical difference between the mathematical 'sciences' and others; but for my present purpose this hardly matters.

its laws of refraction, and also the science of chemistry, which became involved because of the importance of the composition of the glass. Nowadays the construction of 'electron-microscopes' also involves the science of nuclear physics. This example also illustrates how it is possible for one science to be replaced by another as the science of paramount importance to a technique. Even where this does not happen, it is the rule and not the exception for a technique to involve more than one science, as modern agriculture, for instance, involves genetics, botany, organic chemistry and to a lesser degree other sciences.

As I shall be referring constantly to techniques and their peculiar features, I had better explain at this stage one or two terms to which I have had to give a special meaning. With quite a number of techniques there is more than one way of achieving the objective of the technique. In the field of egg-production, for example, there is the free-run system, in which the hens are allowed to run about in an enclosed area; there is the battery system, in which each hen spends all her life in a small separate pen; and there is the deep-litter system, in which a large number of hens is kept indoors in a shed. These are what I call 'sub-techniques'—different and alternative sets of rules for attaining the same end. There are also what I call 'intermediate techniques', which are techniques for arriving at some intermediate stage on the way to the ultimate objective. In strategy, for example, military tactics are an intermediate technique for achieving the intermediate objective of winning battles. Sometimes we come across devices or expedients which, though not essential to a technique, are nevertheless used because they enable it to achieve its object with greater speed, efficiency or thoroughness. Thus a smoke-screen or an artillery barrage, though not necessarily essential to a military assault, may greatly increase its efficiency by reducing casualties. Such expedients I propose to call 'facilitants'. Finally, when I use the words 'technician' I am of course referring to the practitioner of a technique as opposed to a scientist; and I shall use 'technical' in the same way.

Quite a few professions and pursuits that like to call themselves sciences are really techniques. Architecture is an obvious example. Another example, which is important for the subject we are going to consider, is medicine. This is not a science, although it makes use of a large number of sciences, among which, to name only a few, are chemistry, physics and biology. Medicine itself, however, even in its broadest sense, is a technique for remedying disorders in living organisms. By 'medicine' we usually mean 'remedial medicine', and this is the sense in which I shall use it in this book; when we want to refer to the technique for preventing disorders we call it 'preventive medicine'. There is, however, one red and rather snobbish herring with which I had better deal at this point. Some practitioners of medicine, realizing that there is some odd quality about it which makes it rather strained to call it a science, but not wanting to detract from its status by calling it a 'craft' or 'technique', have taken to saying that it is an 'art'. They do not mean that its results have any aesthetic value; the word is used, I think, to suggest that medicine, like painting or poetry-writing, achieves its results by means that are known intuitively and are not acquired by a planned curriculum of training. For some reason this is thought to be more meritorious. There are several fallacies here. The first is to suppose that if, as may well be true, you cannot become a good doctor simply by reading books and attending lectures and clinical sessions this means that the essence of doctoring is acquired by intuition. It is much more likely that it is acquired, like a low golf-handicap, by the very ordinary and familiar process of practice—by doing something badly and then doing it better. The second fallacy is to assume that the secret of an artistic achievement lies in the method by which the results are achieved, when it really lies in being able to tell whether the results are good or bad, and whether they should be left alone, improved or scrapped. The methods by which these results are achieved, whether it is the mixing of colours for a painting or the gestures of an actor, are learned, like other techniques, partly from books and lectures and partly from hard practice; and we do in fact refer to the 'technique' of a painter or actor. It is probably true of course that some people are 'natural' actors in the sense that they seem to be able to act well with the minimum of practice; but this happens in all techniques—some people are 'natural' golfers. There is only one sense in which it seems to me proper to call the achievement of an objective an 'art', and that is if you mean simply that it is a technique whose rules are hard to formulate. But in all probability this is a temporary state of affairs. As time goes on, ways are found of formulating more and more rules for more and more techniques which have hitherto been regarded as incommunicable.

5

Psychiatry is of course the technique of remedying or alleviating mental disorders. The group of semantic methods which, as we saw, are grouped together under the heading of 'psychotherapy' are therefore sub-techniques, just as non-semantic methods such as electro-convulsion treatment are also sub-techniques. We shall see later that most, if not all, of the psychotherapeutic sub-techniques involve what I call 'intermediate' techniques for arriving at some particular stage on the way to the ultimate objective. Like the technique of medicine, psychiatry makes use of sciences— chemistry when it is using drugs, electro-physics when it is using electro-convulsions, physiology when it is performing operations on the central nervous system. Like the physical sub-techniques, the psychotherapeutic ones also make use of sciences. Chemistry is involved when drugs such as sodium pentothal or lysergic acid diethylamide are used to assist communication with the patient. But one science is of particular importance to psychotherapy, and that is of course psychology. In fact, the extent to which the psychotherapeutic sub-techniques rely on psychology, to the virtual exclusion of other sciences, makes them somewhat unusual among techniques, and has helped to obscure the important fact that they are not themselves sciences or potential sciences. But the use of drugs by some psychotherapists shows that the technique can make use of other sciences, and that its marriage to psychology is not necessarily monogamous.

All present-day sciences are a mixture of two kinds of statement, in proportions which vary with each science. On the one hand there are statements which either

(a) record observations; for example, 'When I dipped the piece of paper into the liquid, the paper turned blue': or

(b) summarize observations; for example, 'All alkalis turn litmus paper blue.'

These are 'descriptive' statements, or as Toulmin has nicknamed them, 'natural history' statements.[1] Scientific statements of

---

[1] *The Philosophy of Science*, Hutchinson's University Library, 1953.
Very few such statements are as simple as this example from school chemistry. Most of the important 'descriptive' statements of modern science need an advanced mathematical notation to make the summary compact enough to be comprehended. Snell's Law of Refraction, for example, states that 'Whenever any ray of light is incident at the surface which separates two media, it is bent in such a way that the ratio of the

the other kind are 'explanatory'. These do not record or summarize observations: they try to provide explanations for them. These explanations have two functions. They satisfy an intellectual demand for something that will give coherence and intelligibility to a series of otherwise unconnected phenomena:[1] and they enable us to predict other observations in slightly different situations. Imagine two men living on a plain by the banks of a river that sometimes floods the surrounding country. One is a pure observer; he records the dates of each flood, and after a certain amount of data has been collected he is able to remove his cattle and other belongings in time to avoid the seasonal inundations. Occasionally, however, he is caught by a flood that occurs at the wrong time of year. The other man is of a more inquisitive turn of mind, and reasons that all the extra water that makes the river overflow must come from somewhere. It seems to have no connection with the rainfall in the plain where he lives, but it occurs to him that it may be the effect of rainfall in the distant hills. He is therefore able to predict floods not only every autumn but after every thunderstorm on the north-western horizon, and is to that extent a better predictor of floods than his neighbour. What is more, if he moves to a lowland farm in some other country he will not take so long as his neighbour to learn when to expect floods there. This illustrates the difference between observation and explanation. Some scientists, it is true, take the purist view that the aim of every science should be to do without statements of the explanatory kind, and confine itself to recording observations. They quite rightly point out that the intellectual satisfaction which we get out of explaining phenomena is beside the point, and that if our summaries of our observations were in the proper form we should not need explanations to help us to predict other observations, since these would be deducible from the summaries. Explanations involve the unscientific notion of cause, and it should be the aim of every scientist to replace this with an observed correlation.

Fortunately this is a question that we do not have to go too

sine of the angle of incidence to the sine of the angle of refraction is always a constant quantity for these two media'. Sometimes it is not possible to summarize the observations as compactly as this, and the scientist has to resort to tabulation, as for instance in the case of coefficients of expansion.

[1] For a useful analysis of what we expect of an explanation, see *The Explanation of Human Behaviour*, by F. V. Smith, 1951.

deeply into, since we are concerned here not with the ideal science but with sciences as they are (and probably always will be). It is true that there are some sciences that consist very largely of observations and very little of explanations; what used to be called natural history and is now called 'ethology' is an example. Others, such as mathematical physics, seem to consist very largely of explanations. Obviously, too, the less the scientist is able to explain the more he must rely on observation. Babylonian astronomy relied very largely on observation for this reason, whereas modern astronomers, although interested in adding new stars to their maps, are more concerned to perfect their explanations of what they see.

All explanations make use of what are called 'models'. These consist of entities which we use in our thoughts to provide similar explanations for a number of phenomena. If, whenever we see a river rising, we say 'Ah! Rain somewhere', we are using a scientific model of a crude kind. When we explain our ginger cat's tortoiseshell kittens in terms of genes and chromosomes we are also using a model. Models can be of several kinds. They can be what I call 'corresponding'; that is, they can consist of entities that correspond to what we should observe if instead of thinking of explanations we could observe all that was going on. The man who said to himself 'Rain in the hills' when he saw his river rising was using a corresponding model, because his thoughts corresponded to something he could have observed in certain circumstances. The housewives, on the other hand, who blamed the fairies when their milk turned sour were almost certainly using a non-corresponding model. Some models are actually invented before they are observed to be corresponding: the chromosomes of genetics were assumed to exist before they were observed under the microscope.

It is very important to distinguish a genuine explanatory statement, which uses a model, from the sort of statement which appears to explain but in fact does no more than generalize. The confusion arises because we are in the habit of answering the question 'Why does this happen?' in two quite different ways. If I am asked 'Why does this bar of iron get longer when it is heated?', I can reply 'Because the molecules which make it up move about more violently when it is hot, and take up more room'; and this is a genuine explanation, using a model. But I may also get away with the answer that 'All metals expand when heated' (and I may add a few impressive coefficients of expansion). This is not explaining,

8

however, it merely gives a summary of the observations that have been made of this kind of phenomenon, and shows how the expansion of this bit of iron is simply one instance of many. This is what I shall call 'explaining by summary'. It is intellectually satisfying, but is of less help in predicting the circumstances in which the phenomenon will or will not be repeated.

Some models are 'lifelike'; they resemble phenomena that can be observed in real life. 'Rain in the hills' is a lifelike model. When the Greeks explained storms as the actions of anthropomorphic deities, they were using a lifelike model, although it was a non-corresponding one. Unlifelike models are rarer, since we are forced to invent them only when we cannot use anything we have observed to account for the phenomena we are trying to explain. Perhaps the best examples are the isobaric lines which the meteorologists draw on their weather-maps to show areas of high and low pressure, or the contour lines on topographical maps. The entities of the model of atomic physics began, in the days of Democritus, by being quite like visible particles (Lucretius called them 'semina' or 'seeds') and even in the nineteenth century molecules behaved rather like billiard balls, while atoms were like miniature solar systems. Nowadays physicists think in terms of entities which have been deprived of all their lifelike qualities, and possess only mass, charge and position (and sometimes even their position is doubtful). From the scientific point of view it does not matter how lifelike or unlifelike a model is; what matters is that it should do its job efficiently. The more phenomena it can be used to explain and predict, the more efficient it is. Whether it is corresponding or not is also a secondary question, although not unimportant; for a corresponding model is less likely to mislead you into some incorrect prediction. Perhaps for this reason there is a tendency to think of the model of nuclear physics as the only really trustworthy model, and of all others as to some degree misleading. This can itself be a misleading assumption. It is true that in theory we have no reason to doubt that the model of nuclear physics can be used to explain all possible observations. In practice, however, we shall get better and quicker results in most cases by using some obviously crude and limited model. The dynamics of a child's see-saw, for example, can be handled much more easily if we use the obviously non-corresponding model of the school-books, with arrows to show the direction of forces and so on.

EXPLAINING HUMAN BEHAVIOUR

These distinctions between 'descriptive' and 'explanatory' statements, and this brief account of the role of 'scientific models', are necessarily incomplete and crude. For example, in practice many scientific statements are mixtures of these two kinds, and the distinction between the phenomena and the model is often blurred. But in order to appreciate the true nature of the statements of psychology, and the relationship between the apparently different accounts of behaviour that are offered by the psychologists, it is essential to be able to distinguish between the descriptive and the explanatory elements in a statement, and to detect a model when it is being used. Thinking is a subject which people find it difficult to think about, and even more difficult to talk about, without confusion.

The task of making up 'descriptive' summaries is complicated by the fact that there have always been two kinds of phenomena to choose from—the thoughts, memories and feelings that one can observe in oneself by introspection, and the behaviour that one can observe in other people. The former result in what I have called the 'introspective' description, the latter in the 'behaviourist' kind. One trouble is that it is difficult not to use introspective concepts as explanations for behaviourist descriptions; in other words, to explain what we see people doing by assuming that they are thinking or feeling what we should be thinking or feeling in the circumstances. The result is that introspective words are sometimes genuine descriptions (that is, when they are first-hand accounts of what you or I felt or thought in some situation) but are more often assumed explanations of observed behaviour—that is, are more often used as psychological models.

With the development of the science of physiology, a third kind of description has become fashionable over the last hundred years. It has become possible to observe and measure the changes that take place in various parts of the human mechanism in certain types of situation. It is of course ancient knowledge that our skins sweat and our hearts pound when we know we are in danger. Nowadays, however, we can observe and measure the conductivity of the skin to electric currents, the pulse-rate and pressure of the blood, the secretion of gastric juices and the changes of colour in the lining of the stomach. Most important of all, we can observe and measure activity in the central nervous system, either by observation during brain surgery or by recording changes of electric potential on the electro-encephalograph. As a result we have the physiological type of description which the behaviourist school of psychologists prefer to the introspective, for the very understandable reason that unlike the phenomena of introspection they can be observed by more than one person and can be accurately measured. But like introspective concepts they are also used as explanatory models to account for the behaviour that is described in reflexological terms. It is particularly common to find neurological statements—by which I mean statements about the central nervous system—used like this to explain the way in which a man acts or speaks.

We thus have a situation in psychology in which statements of three kinds are being made—behaviourist, physiological and introspective; of which the first are always descriptive, but the second and third can be used either in descriptive or in explanatory statements. It is, I think, dissatisfaction with this situation that has driven so many twentieth-century psychologists to aim at accounts of human behaviour that are unmistakably descriptive, and, where explanation is demanded, to use concepts that are obviously models, and cannot be mistaken for physiological or phenomenological descriptions. Consider, for example, a situation in which a child is both attracted by sweets which it can see within reach, and held back by a parental ban on sweet-eating; the child can be observed approaching and retreating from the sweets, and perhaps circling round them. To explain this behaviour K. Lewin will draw a diagram in which arrows show the sweets' attraction and other arrows, in the opposite direction, show their repulsion. He may even outline an area within which the repelling 'forces' are stronger than the attracting ones. This topological psychology, as it has been called, is of course strongly reminiscent of the diagrams of school dynamics, with its arrows to represent gravity, momentum, air resistance and so on. The important thing about it, however, is that it is a deliberate attempt to use an explanatory model that is, like the isobars of meteorology, obviously nothing but a model.[1]

While psychologists have been developing in this direction,

[1] Other systems of this kind are described in F. V. Smith's *Explanation of Human Behaviour*, 1951.

considerable progress has been made with the explanatory model of physiology, and particularly neurology. Some of this progress has been the result of experiments with the dead or living brain. Some of it has accompanied the development of the new technique of cybernetics, the study of how machines can be devised to carry out tasks which have hitherto required control by a brain. The design of electronic computers, of automatic aircraft pilots and of 'mechanical tortoises' has shown how the neurons of the brain might be organized so that even its most complex operations could be the result of the same kind of mechanical functioning. They do not of course prove that the brain does work in this way, because they merely offer an analogy; but they show that it would not be impossible for such high-grade tasks as the calculation of cube-roots or the translation of Chinese lyrics into English to be performed by a machine consisting of parts which have been observed in the brain, if these parts were linked up in certain kinds of circuits. All this suggests that the neurological model for the explanation of human behaviour is in all probability a corresponding model.

If so, why should we bother to use any other kind of model? If the explanations of neurology correspond to what is going on in reality, what is the point of using either the deliberately non-corresponding models of the modern psychologists, or the phenomenological explanation in terms of thoughts and feelings that we use in everyday life? The answer to this question is of great importance to a proper understanding of the respective roles of psychology, neurology and psychotherapy.

From the scientific point of view the usefulness of the neurological model is that it links human behaviour to the behaviour of the rest of nature by showing how it can be explained in terms of electro-chemical processes, which in their turn can be explained in terms of the universal model of atomic physics. It is also the best way of explaining why a tumour in a certain area of the brain results in impaired speech, or why meningitis produces certain symptoms. Its limitation is that it does not help us to explain the other 99 per cent of human behaviour: for example, why a child left alone in a room with a box of sweets can be unhappy. We believe that in theory the neurological model could be used to explain this, but in practice it is too complicated to use. It is like the example which I mentioned earlier: trying to use the model of atomic physics to explain the dynamics of a children's seesaw. For the explanation of everyday human behaviour we are forced to resort to one of the other kinds of model, either the deliberately non-corresponding models of the modern behaviourists (such as Lewin) or the time-honoured introspective model which has been used since man first learned to ascribe to other men the same thoughts and feelings as he observed in himself. Without in any way be-littling the efforts of the behaviourists to evolve a scientific model, we must grant that at the present time the introspective model has both greater accuracy and wider utility. We are better at predict-ing other people's actions, and we are more satisfied with our explanations of them, if we simply put ourselves in their place and imagine what we would feel, think and decide.

Quite apart, however, from the scientific point of view, there is the technical standpoint. What does the technician require of a model? Like the scientist he needs one, of course, that will enable him to predict and explain. Unlike the scientist he does not care whether it links up his field with other fields—for example, whether his model is in turn explicable in terms of atomic physics. Nor does he need to worry so much whether his model is a cor-responding one or not; its purpose is to help him to do something —to make or repair or prevent something—and not to provide an explanation that will cover all sorts of unlikely phenomena. But the most important thing that he requires of his explanatory model is that it shall help him to work out what to do to achieve his end. It must offer him a cause that he can manipulate. The maker of optical instruments must be able to think of light as something that he can bend or cut off. That is the main reason why the models of academic psychology are of little use to the technician who wants to be able to alter human behaviour. Those models are not necessarily designed to indicate a cause of behaviour which the technician can attack. Lewin's topological model, for example, does not suggest how the child's behaviour in the presence of the sweets can be altered—unless by removing either child or sweets. This is not a defect in the psychologists' models; it is simply that they are scientists' and not technicians' models.

Technicians whose job is to alter human behaviour use either the neurological or the introspective model. Which they use de-pends on the particular technique on which they are relying. For in techniques as in sciences discoveries are often made first and explained afterwards. In 1835, for example, a suicidally-minded

Belgian tried to kill himself by putting a bullet through his temples. The bullet passed through the frontal lobes of the brain, but instead of dying he became saner. This—and a number of other accidental but similar occurrences[1]—suggested that mental disorders might be cured or alleviated by severing the frontal lobes from the rest of the brain. The effects of this upon the patient's personality, however, were sometimes unfortunate; he often became an animal without foresight or sense of responsibility. Better results were obtained by severing some but not all of the connections between the frontal lobes and the rest of the brain, and this is now an established and valuable technique for alleviating severe cases of certain types of mental disorder. But all this took place without any clear explanation of why the operation should have this effect, and even now the explanations are still very theoretical and vague. It is not only in mental treatment that technical discoveries without explanations are made; not long ago it was found that the growth of pigs could be improved by putting penicillin in their food; but nobody knew why. Sometimes, of course, the explanatory model does suggest a new technique. The knowledge that the brain functioned by means of electro-chemical changes in its neurons suggested the idea of passing a current through it to see whether this would alleviate certain disorders—such as depressive states; and it worked. The result was what is known as electro-convulsion therapy. But even here it is far from clear why this expedient should have worked. The explanation, of course, hardly matters (except from the point of view of one's intellectual satisfaction) if the technique is 100 per cent successful. But few techniques are, and the technicians' chances of improving on their methods are obviously greatly increased if they are using an explanatory model that suggests what may be wrong in the unsuccessful cases or what variations on the method should be tried.

In the development of psychotherapy there are quite a few points at which technical discovery has preceded explanation in this way. There are of course instances, as we shall see, of theoretical explanations in their turn suggesting further technical innovations, and when we are considering some elaboration of psychotherapeutic theory it will be useful to ask whether it did in fact contribute any important change to the technique. It will be easier to answer this question if we appreciate that in the psychotherapeutic tech-

[1] See *Personality and the Frontal Lobes*, by Asenath Petrie, 1953.

nique such changes may be of two main kinds. They may be changes of *method*; a psychotherapist may decide to do less talking himself and make the patient do more, or to encourage the patient to do more remembering and less phantasying. Changes of this kind can amount to the introduction of a new *intermediate technique*. On the other hand they may be changes of *topic*; the psychotherapist may decide that it will be profitable to concentrate the conversation on sexual matters, or on the patient's aggressive impulses. So that in order to be clear about the differences between two *sub-techniques*—such as those of Freud and Jung—it is useful to try to sort them into

(i) differences of *method* amounting to new *intermediate techniques*;
(ii) differences of *method* not amounting to new intermediate techniques;
(iii) differences of *topic*;
(iv) differences in the *explanatory model* which do not really lead to (i), (ii) or (iii).

I have devoted what may seem too large a section of such a short book to these logical prolegomena. But for the rest of this book the reader will be thinking about different ways of thinking about the way in which people think, and many discussions between different psychotherapeutic schools have convinced me of the need for an adequate logical language in which such discussions can be carried on.

Recommended Reading

THE PHILOSOPHY OF SCIENCE, by Stephen Toulmin. Hutchinson's University Library, 1953.
THE EXPLANATION OF HUMAN BEHAVIOUR, by F. V. Smith. Constable, 1951.

II

PRIMITIVE PSYCHOANALYSIS

FREUD

SIGMUND FREUD (1856–1939), the ultimate source of all but one of the modern schools of psychotherapy, achieved this position because he was two rare things at once. He was, as it were, the meeting-point of several distinct intellectual approaches to the problem of neurotic disorders, and at the same time a technician who, having discovered an effective technique, was ready to modify it time and again to fit new observations and ideas.

In the first place, Freud was a Jew, as so many psychoanalysts have been since. Although he was a free-thinker and not a practising Jew in the religious sense, it is interesting to speculate how much his contribution to modern thought owes to the Hebraic tradition and inheritance. The Jewish religion, for example, threw open its arcana to reason and the free play of intellect many generations before Christianity did so; and in the Middle Ages it was the Jewish philosophers who reconciled the Christian monks to the ideas of Aristotle. This tradition may have helped Freud to think scientifically and dispassionately about matters which, then as now, were disturbing to the moral sense, and not least his own. At the same time, it is also part of the Hebraic tradition to avoid anthropomorphism, and to deny the ability of any one intellect to comprehend God or the universe. Léon Roth has pointed out[1] how, in the same half-century, Bergson, Alexander, Freud and Einstein have all in their way 'set the human intellect in its place'. Freud's determinism, too, his insistence on tracing all mental phenomena to past causes, is consistent with the Jewish suspicion of doctrines which profess to descry the final purpose of man or the world. He shared, too, the Jew's capacity not only for introspection

[1] In *The Legacy of Israel*, 1927.

16

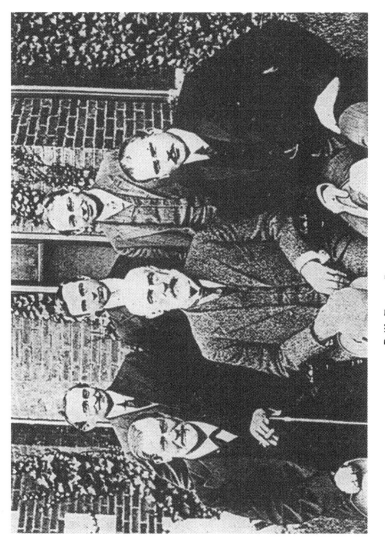

Brill, Ernest Jones, Ferenczi,
Freud, Stanley Hall, and Jung
at Worcester College, Massachusetts in 1909.

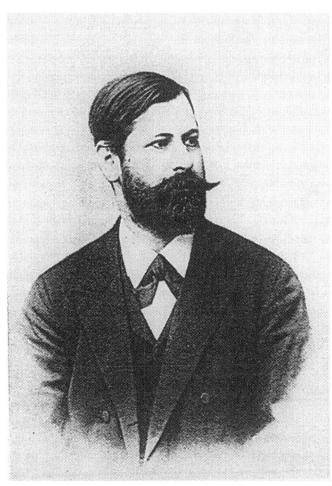

Freud, aged thirty-five.

[to face page 16

but also for using its results to guess the thoughts and feelings of others—a capacity which may have had survival value in the evolution of this persecuted race. He once remarked that to be unable to divine someone else's thoughts gave him an uncanny feeling.

Nor must it be overlooked that Freud himself suffered from one variety of the neuroses that he treated. During the period when he was developing his own technique he experienced excessive anxieties about death and fears of long journeys; he alternated between moods of elation and depression; he suffered from cardiac and gastric troubles with no determinable physical cause. (His brothers and sisters also suffered from symptoms that he described as 'hysterical'.) These symptoms must have given him not only sympathy with but also insight into the neurotic's ways of thinking and behaving.[1]

Freud spent practically the whole of his working life in Vienna. He received his schooling at the Gymnasium, where he received the usual thorough grounding in the classics, and in the sixth form made the acquaintance of academic psychology in the form of a text-book written by a follower of Herbart; the importance of this will become clearer later. At the University, however, he became a medical student. It is clear that he did so not because of any desire to practise medicine (which he did his best to avoid) but because of an interest in physiological research. He took three years more than was necessary to acquire his medical degree, largely because he spent most of the time in the physiological laboratory of Brücke. Gradually his interest gravitated—or was steered by Brücke—in the direction of the nervous system, and his first paper on this subject was published when he was only twenty-one. Even when he at last took his medical degree it was only in order to qualify himself for a career in the teaching of physiology, and it was not until Brücke warned him that his lack of private means made this out of the question that he finally, in 1882 at the age of twenty-six, entered hospital as a Clinical Assistant. Six months of his first year were spent in the Psychiatric Department of the great Meynert. Freud's interest in the physiology of the nervous system had now begun to concentrate on the human brain,

---

[1] It will be obvious how much I owe in this chapter to the first volume of the painstaking biography of Dr. Ernest Jones, who has recorded the ascertainable facts, whether important or trivial, but has wisely left it to others to assess their significance.

and his chief was so impressed by some of Freud's published researches that he offered to hand over his lecturing work to him; but Freud refused. For purely financial reasons (as he himself emphasizes) he now began to study diseases of the human central nervous system, a subject in which few Viennese doctors specialized. He published a number of papers on this subject, and became so expert at diagnosing the site of damage to the brain that his lectures were attended even by students from America.

Although useful progress was being made at this period in tracing disorders to physical damage to different parts of the nervous system, this process was occasionally carried too far. Freud himself made fun of his own expertise in his autobiography:

> I understood nothing about the neuroses. On one occasion I introduced to my audience a neurotic suffering from a persistent headache as a case of chronic localized meningitis; they quite rightly rose in revolt against me and my premature activities as a teacher came to an end. By way of excuse I may add that this happened at a time when greater authorities than myself were in the habit of diagnosing neurasthenia as cerebral tumour.[1]

Even the post-mortem researches of the dissecting-rooms were not suggesting any very effective means of treating disorders of the nervous system. In cases of neurasthenia,[2] for example, the physician of the day could prescribe rest, preferably in a spa, with massage, baths and electrical stimulation of the muscles. Freud himself used these prescriptions in his early private practice.

HYPNOTISM

He had, however, some acquaintance with a totally different method of treating these unsatisfactory disorders. About a hundred years before, Anton Mesmer (1734–1815), another Viennese doctor, had begun to take an interest in the comparatively new study of magnetic phenomena. One of the inmates of his house was a woman of twenty-nine, a Miss Oesterline, who suffered

---

[1] *An Autobiographical Study*, 1925.
[2] A group of symptoms, of which the chief is chronic lassitude, accompanied by inability to concentrate and sometimes hypochondria and depression. As its name indicates, it was for a long time ascribed to a literal 'weakness of the nerves'.

periodically from 'blood rushing to the head, toothache and ear-
ache, followed by delirium, rage, vomiting and swooning' but was
relieved after these attacks had reached 'beneficial crises'.[1] He
applied three pieces of magnetized iron to her stomach and legs,
whereupon she felt 'painful currents of a subtle material which
. . . made their way towards the lower part and caused all the
symptoms of the attack to cease after six hours'.[1] He moved to
Paris and developed this method into an impressive procedure. He
would make his patient sit with her back to the north; to the
accompaniment of soothing music he would press the pit of her
stomach and make passes in front of her face, meanwhile staring
into her eyes. Sometimes he seated his subjects against 'magnetized' trees, or round a tub containing water and iron filings, from
which he told them that the 'magnetic fluid' emanated. His subjects would fall into a trance, sometimes called 'mesmeric sleep',
during which he would tell them that their symptoms would disappear. At first he attributed his results to 'magnetism' but when
he discovered that he could achieve them merely by touching the
patient with his fingers, he decided that there was an influence
which he called 'animal magnetism', and which could be com-
municated to inanimate objects. The controversy that at once arose
led to the appointment of three successive Commissions by the
French scientists, in 1784, 1825 and 1831. The first found that the
same results could be achieved if the patient were deceived into
believing herself[2] to be in the vicinity of one of Mesmer's 'magnetized objects', while no results were achieved if she were in its
vicinity and did not know it; and they concluded that 'the imagination does everything, the magnetism nothing'. As the second Com-
mission realized, this did not affect the genuineness of the cures,
although it did show the inadequacy of Mesmer's explanatory
model. But partly on these fallacious grounds, partly because of
the ambitious claims of the mesmerists to be able to cure a wide
variety of disorders, his methods fell into discredit. By about 1840,
however, demonstrations of it by Frenchmen had aroused the
interest of English doctors such as Eliotson and Esdaile, who

[1] *Mémoire sur la découverte du Magnetisme Animale*, by A. Mesmer,
1779, tr. V. R. Myers, 1948.
[2] Throughout this book I shall refer to the practitioner as 'he' and to
the patient as 'she', in order to avoid any ambiguous pronouns. It is in
any case worth noting that in the first examples of psychotherapy recorded
by Mesmer, Breuer, Freud and Jung, the patients were women.

found it an excellent means of anaesthetizing patients for surgery.[1] 'Mesmeric clinics' for the treatment of disorders were set up in London, Edinburgh, Dublin and elsewhere.

The discredited magnetic explanation had by now been replaced by a neurological model, which accounted for the phenomena in terms of the fatigue of the sensory nerves; but Braid, a Manchester physician, had realized that a better explanation could be devised in terms of 'ideas'—that is, what I called in the previous chapter an 'introspective' model. He thought that the patient was in a sort of sleep, which he called 'hypnosis'; his method of producing this state was to make her gaze fixedly at some small bright object, and he therefore concluded that the essential factor was a narrowing of the attention, which he called 'monoideism', meaning 'concentration on one idea'. This fitted in well with a prevalent nineteenth-century view of mental activity as consisting of a collection of 'ideas', which interacted according to more or less mechanical laws. One idea could be expelled from the mind by another contradictory idea. They could have properties just as material objects did, and could be pleasant or unpleasant, vague or vivid. They were in fact a mental counterpart of the atoms of which Dalton had recently shown the physical world to consist. The most thorough and elaborate model on these lines had just been worked out by the German psychologist and educationalist Herbart, and was the basis of the text-book which Freud had used in the sixth form at school.

Braid's theory of hypnotism was eagerly taken up in France. At Nancy the French physician Liébeault (1823–1904) founded a clinic where he treated physical disorders by hypnotizing his patients and then telling them that their symptoms would disappear. As we shall see in Chapter VIII it is from Liébeault's method of 'hypnotic suggestion' that the modern suggestive school is descended. In Paris the neurologist Charcot (1825–1913) used hypnotized hysterics for his famous demonstrations, which drew audiences from most of the countries of the western world.

---

[1] This use of hypnotism went out of fashion only because of the invention of anaesthesia by chloroform and other drugs, and it is only recently that its advantages over these in normal childbirth, dentistry and some surgical operations have begun to be recognized.

FREUD AND HYPNOTISM

Hypnotic suggestion was by no means unknown in Vienna when Freud began to study medicine. As a student he attended demonstrations by a hypnotist called Hansen. These demonstrations were also witnessed by Benedikt, the chief of the Vienna Policlinic, and by a family doctor called Joseph Breuer. Benedikt was a widely-travelled and broadminded physician, whose interests included phrenology and anthropology as well as hypnotism, and in 1878 at congress in Paris he was impressed by Charcot's demonstrations. (Later, in 1894, he himself published a book called *Hypnotism and Suggestion*.) Freud was undoubtedly influenced by Benedikt, and when in 1885 he was awarded a travelling grant it was Benedikt who gave him an introduction to Charcot.[1]

He was even more strongly influenced, however, by Breuer, who took a fatherly interest in his career and helped him with generous loans. From December 1880 to June 1882 Breuer treated a twenty-one-year-old girl called Bertha Pappenheim, whose symptoms were paralysis of three limbs, with contractures and anaesthesias, disturbances of sight and speech, inability to eat and a nervous cough. She was also a case of dual personality, and in the transition from one to the other she entered a 'hypnoid state', during which she would talk to Breuer about her symptoms. This seemed to give her temporary relief, and was encouraged by Breuer. One day she told him the details of the first appearance of one particular symptom, and to the astonishment of physician and patient it disappeared. Breuer, who was sufficiently interested to visit her every day for over a year, made her go through this process with each of her symptoms, and as her spontaneous hypnoid states were either too short or inconveniently timed he took to inducing them artificially by hypnosis. He called this method 'catharsis'—that is, 'purging'. Miss Pappenheim called it, more literally, 'the talking cure'.

Breuer told Freud about the success[2] of this method. What he

---

[1] A few months before leaving for Paris, Freud gained more experience of hypnotism when he worked for a short time at a private psychiatric sanatorium where hypnotic suggestion was practised by the superintendent, Leidesdorf.

[2] Its success was rather temporary, since Miss Pappenheim had subsequent relapses. Ernest Jones' biography (vol. I, p. 247) gives the rest of her story.

did not tell him until later was that the patient became embarrassingly attached to her physician as a result of it.

At the Salpêtrière Freud found hypnotism used not as a means of therapy but as an instrument for scientific study. Charcot, who incidentally never hypnotized anyone himself but left this to his assistants,[1] took a neurologist's interest in the phenomena of hysteria. This was a generic name for various combinations of tremors, tics, convulsions, paralyses, anaesthesia, fainting-fits and vomiting, which seem to have been almost an occupational disorder of Victorian womanhood. Since the time of Hippocrates it had been attributed to a disordered womb, whence its name; but it can only have been this preconceived theory which prevented it from being observed in men, although they seem to be less prone to obvious forms of it (except under great stress, such as battle). Charcot not only produced male hysterics, but also showed how the symptoms of hysteria could be produced in both men and women by hypnotic suggestion. He pointed out, too, how in hysterical anaesthesia of, say, the hand, the area of skin that had lost sensation corresponded not to the area that would have been deprived of it by damage to a sensory nerve, but simply to the patient's *idea* of her hand (this is known as the phenomenon of 'glove anaesthesia'). Finally, he demonstrated cases in which symptoms had appeared after an incident that had not damaged the patient physically, but had affected her emotionally.

Charcot's influence on Freud, however, has been overestimated.[2] He did not teach him to treat disorder by hypnotic suggestion; for Freud had already seen this done in Vienna, and in any case Charcot was more interested in creating symptoms for experimental purposes than in removing them. Freud told Charcot about Breuer's cathartic cure, but could not interest him in it. It was Liébeault and his assistant Bernheim (1837–1919) at Nancy who used hypnosis for therapeutic purposes (see Chapter VIII), and Freud soon realized that they had more to teach him than Charcot. In at least one respect Charcot temporarily misled Freud, by asserting that only hysterics could be hypnotized, whereas the

[1] *La Psychologie Contemporaine*, by P. Foulquié and G. Deledalle, 1951. Most of Charcot's experiments and demonstrations were carried out on three female hysterics.

[2] For example by P. Janet, who wrote, 'Le point de départ du Freudisme c'est le séjour de Freud à la Salpêtrière . . .', in the *Journal de Psychologie*, 1923.

Nancy physicians knew very well that other types of patient could be.

Thanks to the work of Professor C. L. Hull, the United States behaviourist,[1] and later experimenters we now have more established facts about hypnosis than the nineteenth-century physicians. For example, the hypnotic trance differs physiologically from sleep[2] in several ways, and also from the state of immobility which can be artificially induced in some animals. With varying difficulty and in different degrees almost all human beings can be hypnotized, the only predictable exceptions being mental defectives, severe cases of schizophrenia and infants who are not old enough to converse—in other words, people with whom it is very hard to communicate. Some experiments suggest that there are certain categories who are slightly more susceptible than most to hypnosis—women, children and the intelligent, amiable or neurasthenic of both sexes.

The technique of hypnotizing need not be as spectacular as Mesmer's. For medical or experimental purposes Braid's method is most often used. The subject is usually made to lie on her back on a couch in quiet surroundings without distractions. She is asked to concentrate her gaze on some small bright object just above the comfortable line of vision, and to relax. The hypnotist tells her that her eyelids are becoming tired and heavy (as in fact they are, for physiological reasons); since she finds that this is so, she comes to accept his statement that she cannot open them (except when he tells her to). He then tells her that her arm is becoming heavy, and in the same way suggests to her that she cannot lift it—unless he tells her to. In this way he suggests to her that without his instructions she can only remain relaxed, but that she can do what he tells her to. With subjects who are susceptible, or who have been hypnotized before, it is often unnecessary to use devices such as the small bright object, and the hypnotic state can be induced simply by instructions to relax, followed by the usual suggestions of drowsiness, heaviness in the limbs and so on. Although stage hypnotists still employ some of the more spectacular devices, the essential feature of all methods of hypnosis seems to be suggestion. Most hypnotists are men, but some have been women; I cannot find any record of a child hypnotist.

[1] See his book *Hypnosis and Suggestibility*, 1933.
[2] Although a hypnotized person can be made to pass into sleep.

Contrary to common belief, the hypnotic state wears off naturally in quite a short time, although it can be terminated more speedily by the hypnotist—or indeed by suggestions from anyone else. The notion that the hypnotized subject can hear and obey only the hypnotist is true only where the hypnotist has given instructions of this sort. On the other hand subjects who are hypnotized frequently by the same person tend to become attached to and dependent on him.

In light hypnosis it is possible to induce artificial paralysis or rigidity of selected limbs, and artificial insensibility to pain in selected parts of the body. Under deeper hypnosis the subject can be made to perform absurd actions, recall memories with exceptional vividness, or forget them, and to see, hear or smell things that are not there; with more difficulty she can be induced not to perceive things that *are* there. (But the belief that hypnosis can produce abnormally acute perception, or an abnormally accurate judgment of time, has not been confirmed.) During hypnosis the subject can be given instructions which she will obey in the post-hypnotic state—for example, to perform absurd actions, forget incidents or even, in some cases, have hallucinations. Hull came to the conclusion that all these effects could be produced by suggestion alone, without hypnosis, although in a much less marked degree; from this point of view the hypnotic state could be regarded as one of 'hyper-suggestibility'. This does not of course mean that it may not have other characteristics; but from the therapeutic point of view the way in which it facilitates suggestion is undoubtedly the most important.

For psychotherapeutic purposes, as we have seen, two hypnotic sub-techniques had been evolved by the time of Freud's visit to France in 1885. Liébeault's method was to tell the hypnotized patient that her symptoms would disappear; this was the sub-technique of 'hypnotic suggestion'.[1] Breuer had achieved results, on the other hand, by inducing the hypnotized patient to recall incidents connected with her symptoms which she was normally unable to recall; this is the sub-technique of 'hypnotic anamnesis'. In both cases hypnosis was at first believed to be essential to the sub-technique, but was soon proved to be merely what I have called in Chapter I a 'facilitant'.

[1] That is, using suggestion upon the hypnotized patient. This must not be confused with the use of suggestion to *induce* hypnosis, which seems to be common to all hypnotic sub-techniques.

THE CONCENTRATION SUB-TECHNIQUE

After Freud's return to Vienna he set up in private practice. For a short while he continued to treat hysteria by prescribing the old remedies of rest, massage, hydrotherapy or electrical stimulation for hysterical disorders. But by the end of 1887 he had adopted hypnotic suggestion, and in May 1889 he also began to use Breuer's hypnotic catharsis. At first he revelled in their success with hitherto intractable cases, but it was not long before he became dissatisfied. In the first place, he soon had to acknowledge that as a hypnotist he was only mediocre. In some patients he could induce only a light hypnosis; some he could not hypnotize at all. In 1889 he paid a visit to the great Bernheim at Nancy (whose book on the hypnotic technique he had translated into German) and found that even he had the same limitations. But there were two other drawbacks. One was that 'even the most brilliant results were liable to be wiped away if my personal relations with the patient became disturbed'. True, the improvement could be restored if there were a reconciliation. But he was suspicious of the extent to which the cure seemed to depend upon the emotional relationship between doctor and patient. He was essentially a prudish and rigidly monogamous man, and like Breuer he was shocked one day when a female patient whom he was awakening from hypnosis flung her arms affectionately round his neck. The third disadvantage was that if the symptoms were to be permanently removed it seemed to be necessary for the patient to be able to recall in waking life what she had recalled under hypnosis; but if the hypnosis had been a deep one, she was often unable to do this. The difficulty was that some patients could recall some incidents only if the hypnosis were a deep one. Bernheim showed him a way out of this difficulty. He insisted that the memory in question was still there, and after the patient had emerged from hypnosis he would tell her that when he laid his hand on her forehead the memory would return. Gradually at first, but eventually 'in a flood and with complete clarity' it did so.

PRIMITIVE PSYCHOANALYSIS

This trick not only helped Freud over this particular difficulty; it also showed him how to dispense with hypnosis altogether. In

1892 he began to use the following technique. He would make his patient lie on a couch as before, but instead of bending over her, face to face, he would sit behind her, out of sight.[1] He would then tell the patient to concentrate upon remembering the incidents connected with the first appearance of her symptoms, and if she had difficulty in doing so he would tell her that when he laid his hand upon her forehead the memories would come into her mind. This seemed to 'facilitate' recall in much the same way as hypnosis, and it put much less strain upon the doctor. I shall refer to it as the intermediate technique of 'concentration anamnesis'—that is, of recall facilitated by concentration. Freud now used hypnotic suggestion—the other hypnotic sub-technique—far less, and by 1896 he had completely abandoned hypnosis. In that year, as Ernest Jones points out, he used the term 'psychoanalysis' for the first time to describe his technique.

We have now reached what can be called the 'primitive phase' of psychoanalysis, which extends until 1897. So far I have described only the development of the technical skeleton, in order that the structure and growth of this should be seen as clearly as possible. It is now time to put a little flesh on the skeleton. But here again I shall try to keep two things separate, for the good reason that a real understanding of the subsequent history of psychotherapy depends upon a clear appreciation of the logical difference between them. I shall describe the observations that Freud made when he was developing his technique; they make up what I called in the previous chapter 'the natural history' of the subject. At the same time I shall try at each stage to show their effect upon the model that Freud used in thinking about his technique.

EFFECT OF THE PAST

One of the most striking things about hypnotic anamnesis or concentration anamnesis was of course the way in which long-past incidents appeared to be connected with present symptoms. The same phenomenon is of course encountered in physical medicine.

[1] He preserved this arrangement throughout the rest of his career, partly because he thought that his patients could think and talk more freely if they could not see him, but chiefly because he himself could not bear to be stared at all day.

A patient who complains of pain in the region of the lower oesophagus will almost certainly be asked by his doctor 'When did you first feel this pain?' He may then reply 'Soon after my Christmas dinner'. But the doctor's mind will not be content with this; he will try to think of some way in which the patient's Christmas dinner can have had an effect upon the patient's present structure which could be causing pain. His knowledge of the rites of Christendom will readily suggest an explanatory model—the presence of a coin or one of the other metallic foreign bodies which are introduced into the Christmas pudding.

Science bases its thinking on one or two general principles. One of these is the principle of 'no action at a distance', which compels us to bridge the gap of ninety-three million miles between sunspots and terrestrial storms with a model of waves or quanta passing through empty space. Another principle, which is less familiar because it seems too obvious to need stating, is the principle of 'no action at a distance in time'. If a milk jug that is dropped on Tuesday comes apart on Friday, science refuses to think of Tuesday's accident as the direct cause of Friday's breakage; the gap must be bridged by assuming a structural defect created by the accident.

If a human being's present behaviour is obviously affected by something that happened in the past, we normally bridge the gap in one of two ways. We may say 'Yes, he remembers what happened last time'; or, if the past incidents are very numerous and not striking enough to be remembered, we talk about 'the acquisition of habits', or about 'practice making perfect'. We thus use the concept of 'memory' or 'habit' as if it were a structural feature of the present state of the person.

Freud was faced, however, with a phenomenon that fitted into neither of these descriptions. His technique consisted of alleviating symptoms by reviving memories of certain incidents. But these memories could be made to appear only by very specialized means, and could not therefore be thought of as a structural part of the present state of their owner's mind. And yet it was essential to think of them in this way, for his technique was enabling him to attack the effect of a past incident, and he could not violate the scientific canon by thinking of himself as manipulating the past.

THE MODEL OF THE UNCONSCIOUS

He found the solution in the Herbartian psychology which he had learned in the sixth form at school. The French school talked in terms of 'ideas' which could be implanted in or removed from the mind of the patient by suggestion. Herbart had similarly treated ideas as if they were material objects—mental atoms that interacted according to his elaborate mathematical laws. But according to Herbart they also resembled atoms in being indestructible. If I think of my breakfast and then cease to do so my idea of breakfast has not ceased to exist, he thought; it has merely been pushed aside by whatever idea subsequently took its place. When I think of my breakfast for the second time, it is because this idea has re-entered consciousness.

Freud found this a very convenient model. It not only explained very well the way in which thoughts can occupy the forefront of our consciousness, can recede into the background (which he called the preconscious) and can be summoned forth again; it also enabled him to describe the status of those memories which could not be summoned up at will but required a special technique for their resuscitation. They were in a third place—the unconscious—from which they were not free to emerge as preconscious ideas did.

This, then, is the logical status of the Freudian concept of the unconscious.[1] More controversy has raged round this than round any other psychological or psychotherapeutic notion—even Freud's notions on the subject of sex. Sceptics, who include both philosophers and academic psychologists, have attacked 'unconscious thoughts' as a contradiction in terms. Mystics have personified the unconscious into a sort of devil, with the difference that it cannot be cast out, but only given a little healthy exercise. Freud himself tried to justify it by using four separate arguments to prove that it existed; they can be studied in his essay, 'The Unconscious' (1915). Briefly, he argued that it could be inferred in the same way as we infer the existence of other people's minds; that without it the chain of conscious mental events became merely an unintelligible, disconnected procession; that his technique showed that

[1] This is the accepted translation of '*das unbewusste*'. The term 'subconscious' was coined by Morton Prince, the American psychologist and hypnotist, to describe the submerged personalities in cases of multiple personality, but is not nowadays used in psychoanalytic literature.

it was the cause of conscious thoughts and behaviour and must therefore be as real as its effects; and that it enabled him to achieve cures. Only one of these arguments will really stand up to a close logical examination.[1] That is the last, which I call the 'argument from results'. This is exactly what one would expect if one were dealing with a scientific or technical model. It would of course be interesting to know whether it is a corresponding model or not; if so, it might prove to have wider and unexpected uses. But the point of it for the scientist or technician is that it works; it lets the scientist predict or the technician work out ways of doing what he wants with his material. The Freudian model is not a scientists' model; it is not of much use for predicting what someone will do in certain circumstances (it is better than psychologists' models, but not so good as our rather vague, intuitive, everyday way of guessing what people will do). It is a technician's model, and allows the technician to think about what he must do in order to achieve his cure. It is rather like an archaeologist's transparent map which he can lay on top of the physical map of the present features of the ground. It does not really show him what is there today; it shows long-vanished Neolithic settlements and battle-fields. But it also tells him where to dig if he wants to find stone axes or burial places. In much the same way the unconscious is an extension, for technical purposes, of the introspective model which we use to explain people's actions when we talk of their 'feelings', 'motives', 'thoughts', 'desires' and so forth.

REPRESSION

All this, of course, did not explain why certain memories should have acquired this peculiar status. Freud observed, however, that those which he succeeded in reviving in this way had certain pro-perties in common. One of these properties was the distress which they caused to their owner. Obviously, therefore, the conscious mind expelled them for this reason.

RESISTANCE

Once expelled, however, they did not 'stay put'. This was clear from another observation, which was that the patient actually

[1] They are discussed in detail in my thesis 'The Logical Status of the Freudian Unconscious' (Edinburgh University Library).

resisted the technician's efforts to bring them back into consciousness: a phenomenon which Freud called 'resistance'. He therefore
visualized repression not only as an initial act of expulsion, but
also as a constant force exercised upon these particular ideas by
the conscious mind. Here again it is striking how mechanistic his
model was.

FREE ASSOCIATION

The phenomenon of resistance led Freud to cast about for other
facilitants to supplement the trick of 'the hand on the forehead'
in reviving the repressed ideas. Apart from direct and systematic
questioning, which was not very successful, he devised two others.
One was 'free association'.[1] Sometimes the thoughts produced by
the patient as a result of the hand on the forehead had no apparent
connection either with the symptom or with the memory which
eventually proved to have a connection with the symptom. Freud
found, however, that if he told the patient to tell him whatever
came into her head, without holding back anything because it
seemed irrelevant or embarrassing, the sequence of thoughts eventually led to ideas that had a clear connection with the symptom.
This curious observation was another thing that could be more
easily visualized by using the spatial, mechanistic model of the
unconscious. For in free association you appear to have an un-
winding, as it were, of the chain of cause and effect. Each idea
leads on to the one which, on Freud's theory, caused it. It is like
a string of objects linked together in such a way that whichever
end you pull the rest come to light.

EMOTIONS

Another important observation which he made was that the revival of a memory had no therapeutic effect unless it was accompanied by the strong and distressing emotions that had accompanied the original experience. He called this 'affective abreaction'
and explained it by saying that the ideas which made up the
memory had a charge of electrical energy (a 'cathexis') which they
could discharge only when they were in the conscious state. It was

---

[1] The other facilitant (dream-interpretation) was not devised until later
(see Chapter III).

this energy which, deprived of its normal outlet because of the repression of the ideas into unconsciousness, had to find abnormal outlets, which might take the form of 'hysterical' symptoms. Consequently Freud's first theory of the reason why his technique alleviated these symptoms was based on Breuer's 'cathartic' theory. Just as Aristotle (who they had no doubt studied at school) thought that drama was good for the audience because it brought about a purge (catharsis) of such emotions as pity and terror, so they thought that this technique purged the patient of the emotions that were 'locked up' along with the unconscious ideas.[1] There is also an obvious analogy between the effect of foreign bodies in the alimentary tract and what he thought of as the effect of ideas in the wrong place.

TRAUMATA

It will be clear from what I have said so far that Freud believed that hysterical disorders could be traced back to particular incidents, the experiencing of which had roused such painful emotions that the patient had had to 'repress' the memory of them. He called such an incident a 'trauma' (which in Greek means 'wound') or sometimes a 'traumatic incident'. The analogy with physical injuries is obvious.

SEXUALITY

Although Charcot had demolished the ancient theory that hysterical symptoms were caused by disorders of the womb, he still believed that there was a close connection between them and sexual activity. In his public utterances he was careful not to stress this, but in private to his students he was franker. '*C'est toujours la chose genitale, toujours, toujours!*' Freud was given much the same advice by Breuer and also by Chrobak, the Viennese gynaecologist, although they afterwards denied this. What led these men to make these statements? In the first place, almost all the hysterical patients whom they saw were women; Freud had great difficulty in finding a case of male hysteria with which to convince his Viennese

---

[1] Later he had some rather pedantic philosophical doubts about the propriety of the notion of 'unfelt feelings'; but he never really abandoned it, although he made it more complicated.

colleagues that such a thing was possible. We know that the sex-distribution of some of the disorders which are connected with psychological factors has changed since then; gastric ulcer, for example, was a woman's complaint in the late nineteenth century and is now common in men and rare in women. It is possible that there has been a similar shift (though not so marked) in the sex-distribution of 'hysteria', and that it really was rare among the males of nineteenth-century Europe. However that may be, there is no doubt that almost all the hysterical patients with whom Breuer, Charcot and Chrobak were concerned were women. Whatever romantic pictures have been painted of nineteenth-century Vienna, the moral and religious codes of that era subjected women to severe sexual disabilities. It was in this generation that an English doctor proclaimed that the suggestion that women could have sexual feelings 'can now be dismissed as a foul asper-sion'. This is perhaps an extreme rather than a typical example of the state of medical knowledge; but there is no doubt that the upper- and middle-class code of the day did not tolerate any free-dom of speech or action by women in sexual matters. A woman with an impotent husband, for example, was prevented by her religious code from seeking divorce, and by her moral code from taking refuge in extra-marital relations. It is therefore quite prob-able that a high proportion of the women who consulted the Viennese or Parisian specialists were in fact suffering from a lack of normal sexual intercourse.

Freud himself was an extremely respectable and almost prudish man (even his most licentious jokes avoided sexual themes), and at the time he regarded his seniors' sayings as no more than the coarse cynicisms of the medical profession.[1] In *Studies on Hysteria* (1895) he said, 'I had come fresh from the school of Charcot, and I regarded the linking of hysteria with the topic of sexuality as a sort of insult—just as the women patients themselves do.' But as

---

[1] Anglo-Saxon readers should not jump to the conclusion that such interests and speculations were confined to a dirty-minded minority of Continental doctors. The Australian doctor, Havelock Ellis, embarked on his gigantic *Studies in the Psychology of Sex* about the same time as Freud began to practise in Vienna, and the first volume was published in 1897. What is more, the mid-nineteenth-century Englishman seems to have had superstitions about the connection between sexual intercourse and good health; Lord Carlisle wrote to a friend, 'I was afraid I was going to have gout the other day. I believe that I live too chaste. It is not a common fault with me.'

he began to specialize himself in the treatment of 'hysterics' by anamnesis he was surprised to find how few of them had had a normal sexual life. Either there was some abnormality in their current sexual life (whether of their own seeking or forced on them by circumstances); or there had been some abnormal sexual incident in their childhood. The former kind of case he called an 'actual neurosis' (because of the toxic effect which he thought misuse of the sexual organs had upon the nervous system); the latter he called a 'psychoneurosis' (because he thought that a psychic entity, the memory of a sexual incident, was causing the disturbance of the nervous system), and this term he (and almost all psychotherapists after him) came to use to denote practically all the disorders which they were called upon to treat.[1] The traumatic incidents which he was able to unearth in all his psychoneurotic cases were sexual experiences occurring at an abnormally early age—that is, before puberty and usually before the age of five. By means of his technique the patient was induced to recall that she had been seduced by some older child or adult.

In its primitive phase, therefore, psychoanalysis was a psychotherapeutic sub-technique which consisted of inducing the patient to recall traumatic incidents from her early childhood. The facilitants used for this purpose were 'concentration' (with or without 'the hand on the forehead') and 'free association'. The traumatic incidents were thought to be sexual seductions by an older child or adult. During this phase Freud did not completely abandon physical methods of treatment. He recommended that the patient undergoing psychoanalysis should also take a 'rest-cure', and sometimes he also advised the 'feeding-up' of the patient.[2]

---

[1] Nobody now believes in an 'actual neurosis' in this sense, and the word 'neurosis' is used as a short equivalent of what Freud called a 'psychoneurosis'. The importance which he attached at this stage to the patient's current sex-life was preserved and later accentuated by followers such as Wilhelm Reich, although orthodox Freudianism had by then ceased to regard it as so important.

[2] *Studies on Hysteria*, 1895. 'Feeding-up' was advocated by the United States psychiatrist, Weir Mitchell, whose book Freud had translated into German in 1887.

Recommended Reading

A HUNDRED YEARS OF PSYCHOLOGY, Pt. I, Ch. VI and Pt. II, Ch. IV, by J. C. Flugel. Duckworth, 1933.

LA PSYCHOLOGIE CONTEMPORAINE, by P. Foulquié and G. Deledalle, pp. 210–15. Presses Universitaires de France, 1951.

AN AUTOBIOGRAPHICAL STUDY, by Sigmund Freud, tr. J. Strachey. Hogarth Press, 1936.

SIGMUND FREUD: LIFE AND WORK, by Ernest Jones. Hogarth Press, 1954 and 1955.

III

LATER FREUDIAN METHODS
A. Interpretation

THE next phase of psychoanalysis began when Freud realized that the seductions which his patients reported were often complete fictions. After he had abandoned hypnosis he had been at pains to avoid 'suggestion', but he still allowed himself to question his patients in a very pressing way. Since he himself was certain that he would eventually unearth a recollection of a childhood seduction, and since he worked under conditions that closely resembled those of the hypnotist, it is not surprising that under his cross-examination his patients soon recalled what he was sure they would recall. Orthodox psychoanalysts ever since have been at the greatest pains to avoid any suspicion of having implanted ideas in the patient by suggestion, and the origin of this taboo lies almost certainly in Freud's uneasy feeling that this was just what he had done in the primitive phase.

Exactly what convinced him that some seduction-memories were fictions is not certain; Ernest Jones guesses that it was one of the results of his own self-analysis, which was proceeding at this time (1897). If so, his reasoning is not so unscientific as it seems at first sight. We have seen that Freud himself undoubtedly suffered from what we should nowadays call neurotic symptoms. If, therefore, he satisfied himself that it was impossible for himself to have suffered in infancy a seduction of the kind he recalled, this provided the single negative instance which is all that is required to falsify a hypothesis. Premature sexual experiences are undoubtedly commoner among children that most adults realize, and tend to be forgotten by the children themselves; but if it is possible to be neurotic without one this cannot be the whole story. And yet, he

35

reasoned, the memories were undeniable phenomena. What was he to think? He concluded that they must be memories not of incidents but of phantasies. But this had startling implications. Children, like women, were supposed to be innocent of sexual feelings (although, as Freud said, every nursemaid knew better). An innocent child can suffer sexual seduction, but to have sexual phantasies a child must have sexual feelings. Was this so?

Between 1889 and 1896 Freud had become the father of three sons and three daughters. Although he was properly reticent about his own family life (an example which not all psychotherapists have followed) his observations of their behaviour must have led him to the conclusion that children far below the age of puberty have sexual interests and desires which, if they are not punished or made to feel guilty, they will gratify in a harmless way. A little later (as a result of his correspondence with Fliess) he decided that between this phase and puberty there intervened the 'latency' period; about the age of seven the child's interest in sex waned and disappeared as a result, Freud thought, of the repression caused by adult disapproval, and did not reappear until puberty.

Freud still retained, therefore, his belief that psychoneurosis had its origin in the sexual life of the child, but now believed that this could consist of 'wishful thinking', and need not necessarily have included actual incidents. His observations of his own children, however, must have shown him that before children took any interest in sexual affairs—for example, in the genitals of themselves or their siblings—they were much more preoccupied with the other orifices—at first the mouth and later the anus. The pleasure they appeared to derive from using or playing with these seemed to be just as absorbing as their later sexual interests. His neurological training reminded him that these three regions—the oral, anal and genital—were those parts of the body which had the highest concentration of sensory nerve-endings; and he knew that all nerves, in whatever part of the body, operated in exactly the same way, by discharges of electrical energy. Thirdly, he seems also to have reasoned that all activity that is not aimed directly at self-preservation is aimed at pleasure, and that pleasure is the same thing whatever the activity (he may also have been influenced by the fact that the German word for pleasure, *lust*, is often used to mean specifically sexual pleasure).

All these arguments probably combined to convince Freud that except in so far as an activity is directly aimed at self-preservation (for example, getting out of the way of a horse) the energy which makes us do it is sexual. He called this energy 'libido' (a nineteenth-century medical term for sexual desire) and he thought that it obeyed the physicists' law of the conservation of energy[1]—that if it were debarred from a direct sexual outlet it would find a way out through some other activity. This kind of energy, together with the instinct of self-preservation, provided the driving force for all human activity. In this way he satisfied his marked desire for simplicity in his theories—for hypotheses that would reduce to the minimum the number of concepts in his model. He was thus trying to apply the excellent principle of Occam's razor— 'don't have any more entities than you must'—just as physicists since Democritus have been trying to reduce matter to the fewest possible kinds of entity.

Even during the phase in which he placed most emphasis on the importance of the sexual group of instincts, Freud recognized that they could not account for all types of human behaviour. At first he recognized a self-preservative instinct as being separate from the sexual ones, but later he decided that this other instinct was that of aggression,[2] and that self-preserving behaviour could be explained as due to self-love, or libido directed towards the self. Freud did not think that the self-preservative instinct could be distorted so as to give rise to neurosis, and it was not until he substituted the notion of aggression that he thought that the source of neurosis could be anything but the sexual instincts.

DEVELOPMENT OF THE PERSONALITY

The model of the unconscious, which in the primitive phase had been merely a repository for repressed memories and their undischarged emotions, was therefore elaborated to include not only the phantasies which Freud had mistaken for memories but also the forbidden urges connected with the mouth, anus and genitals which the infant had been compelled to repress because he was not allowed to satisfy them; it was this bottled-up energy which, in its attempts to discharge itself, found an outlet in curious forms. If

---

[1] Here he was influenced by the experimental psychologist Helmholtz.
[2] Probably under Adler's influence: see Chapter IV.

the individual were fortunate enough in his development the energy was sublimated into socially acceptable activities; he might pursue a Muse instead of a nymph. If he were less fortunate, it issued in 'displaced' forms of pleasure which are less acceptable socially and might even be stigmatized as perversions; for example, sexual pleasure can be derived from unorthodox parts of the body. Alternatively, it might develop into a fear or dislike of the object of the desire, simply because a temptation to which one will not allow oneself to yield is unpleasant. A fourth possibility was that the instinct would be 'turned inward' against its owner. Aggression, for example, can be turned into a self-destructive instinct, and thus result in suicide.

Freud observed that the instinctual development of the child followed certain rules. The unweaned baby was preoccupied with its mouth; this was the oral phase. Later, it passed to an interest in the organs of excretion; this was the anal phase. The third phase was of course the genital phase. But if its transition from one phase to another came under strong prohibition or were for some other reason accompanied by pain instead of pleasure, it might return to an earlier phase. This was called 'regression', and was used to explain the apparent existence among adults of personality types such as the 'oral' (who are preoccupied with the pleasures of the table and seem unaware of those of the bed) or of behaviour patterns such as the 'oral' activities of smoking, sweet-eating or thumb-sucking.[1]

Those were of course aberrations in development. But Freud observed—probably in his own children—other patterns which he thought were universal. The best-known example of these is the 'Oedipus complex'. After the child has entered the genital phase and has begun to feel what we should call sexual feelings in the ordinary sense, it must find an object for them and it seems to select the adult of the opposite sex with whom it has been most closely linked. A boy selects his mother, a girl her father. The very strong taboo on incest makes it necessary for these feelings to be repressed, and in a normal adult they are therefore found only in the unconscious. Freud used this part of his model to explain, for example, why it is that a son who is excessively attached to his

---

[1] Kipling, in the second *Jungle Book* (1895), points out how 'men always play with their mouths', but he would probably not have welcomed any credit for anticipating Freud.

mother (for example, as the result of his father's premature death) tends to marry late in life or not at all.

In this phase of psychoanalysis, therefore, the cause of psychoneurosis was visualized not as a traumatic incident but as a faulty development of the individual's unconscious. Some degree of repression was obviously inevitable if the individual was to form part of a family and later a community; but it was better that a normal desire—whether sexual or aggressive—should be consciously felt and consciously controlled than that it should be allowed no direct expression, and so be forced to assume one of the distorted forms.

Consequently the technique of psychoanalysis ceased to aim at inducing the patient to recall a sexual seduction which had been a traumatic incident in her infancy, and aimed instead at releasing from repression the instincts which had been too severely repressed in infancy. This did not mean that the anamnesis of childhood incidents or phantasies was abandoned; for it was only by recapturing them that the patient could recapture the emotions which they had roused in her and so eventually allow conscious expression to the instincts that had been denied their proper outlet. But it did involve a change in the aim of psychoanalysis, with a consequent development of new intermediate techniques, which in their turn led to new topics and theories.

NEW IDEAS IN TECHNIQUE

Freud was now being very careful to avoid any intermediate technique that might suggest to his patient what she should revive. He would outline to each new patient his theory of how his technique worked, but he would no longer press her to admit something which had not yet occurred to her naturally. He abandoned 'the hand on the forehead', and the only facilitant which he retained from the primitive phase was free association. This was, however, a very severe limitation, and he cast about until he had found two other intermediate techniques with which he could ring the changes when he had temporarily exhausted the possibilities of anamnesis facilitated by free association.

DREAM-INTERPRETATION

Just as the concentration technique had led him to adopt free association as a facilitant, so this in turn led him to the intermediate technique of dream-interpretation. He had always had a strong superstitious interest in dreams; but now he noticed how often the train of thought in free association included the recollection of a dream. During 1897 and for several years afterwards he was engaged in psychoanalysing himself, and by employing free association on the subjects of some of his dreams he found out how to explain them as attempts to fulfil, in phantasy, some wish which he was repressing. Freud's *Interpretation of Dreams*, which appeared in 1900, is his longest and most carefully written continuous work, and it may therefore seem odd to devote so little space to it. But the fact is that, apart from the intrinsic interest of his explanation of this hitherto unintelligible phenomenon, it is for our present purpose merely a thorough exposition of one of his intermediate sub-techniques. This consists of ascertaining the contents of the unconscious by inferences from the features of the dream, the inferences being carried out in accordance with a number of fairly well-defined rules. The best-known of these rules are those of symbolism, by which an idea in the dream is interpreted as representing a different idea in the unconscious. Dream-interpretation was profitable, Freud thought, because in sleep the repressing and censoring part of the conscious mind relaxes its vigilance, and the contents of dreams are therefore more directly determined by the contents of the unconscious than are the contents of our waking thoughts.

INTERPRETATION

Dream-interpretation in its turn led to another intermediate technique. If it is possible to infer the contents of the unconscious from dreams then it must be possible to make similar inferences from our waking thoughts. It is true that these inferences are more difficult and conjectural because our waking thoughts are more subject to repression, and are forced by the conscious, rational mind to 'make sense', so that they are not usually very good material for such inferences. But in the psychoanalyst's consulting-room the patient is schooled to suspend his faculty of censorship as much as possible, particularly when the facilitant of free association is being used, and his thoughts should therefore, Freud reasoned, be one stage nearer to the contents of his unconscious. It might therefore be possible to use some if not all of the rules for dream-interpretation—for example, the rules of symbolism—in order to interpret the waking thoughts of the patient. Freud must have decided that this method yielded results, for he adopted it; and like dream-interpretation it has been one of the standard intermediate techniques of psychoanalysis ever since. Its technical name is simply 'interpretation'.

The new intermediate techniques of interpretation and dream-interpretation had an important effect on the topics which the psychoanalyst discussed with his patient. So long as Freud's only intermediate technique was anamnesis, these topics were necessarily confined to past incidents, feelings and phantasies; but the intermediate techniques of interpretation consisted essentially of inducing the patient to recognize, accept and make conscious her present and not her past desires, attitudes and emotions. It is true that Freud saw and pointed out to his patients the close connection between their present unconscious feelings and those which they were enabled to recall from their childhood by anamnesis. But it also led him eventually to introduce two new topics, whose technical titles are 'the analysis of the transference' and 'ego-analysis'.

TRANSFERENCE

The observation which did more than any other to preserve Freud's belief in the sexual nature of the problem with which he was dealing was the attitude of his patients towards him. I have already mentioned the incident in which one of them embraced him as she was being aroused from the hypnotic state. Other patients, among whom women still predominated, betrayed a similar attraction towards him. Freud explained this by saying that the patient transferred to him the affection which she had felt for some adult (probably the parent of opposite sex) in her childhood. He therefore called this phenomenon 'transference'. As in the primitive phase, he was greatly embarrassed by it, since he regarded it as essentially sexual in nature, and was of course unable to make any response to the patient's desire for a reciprocal affection.[1] It was true that some patients seemed to achieve the

---

[1] In a letter of 1910 to Pfister he says, 'As for the transference it is altogether a curse. . . . The therapeutic result is very good but it is quite dependent on the transference . . .' (Ernest Jones' biography, Vol. II, p. 497).

revival of the past more readily because of their desire to please him and that it could therefore be regarded as a facilitant; but in such cases he found, as he had done with hypnosis, that if the transference towards him disappeared so did the improvement in the patient's condition. He was therefore anxious to avoid what he called the 'cure by love', and tried to abolish the transference by inducing the patient to see it as a symptom having its origin in her childhood; this became a recognized practice, and is known as 'analysing the transference'. It will be clear from what I have said in Chapter I that this was not a new intermediate technique, but an innovation in the topic of the psychoanalyst's conversation with his patient.

It was during this second phase, too, that Freud decided to restrict to the minimum his social contacts with his patients. Hitherto he had seen no harm in entertaining and being entertained by them, and in sharing with them his interests in literature, archaeology or cards. He seems to have come to the conclusion, however, that this interfered with the patient's relationship to him in the consulting-room, which, as we have seen, was beginning to make its importance felt again. If a patient's only contact with her psychoanalyst is in the consulting-room, he can be more or less impersonal in his remarks and manner, and can thus ensure that any reaction of hers is the effect of her neurosis and the transference. It is thus possible, for example, to convince her that any antagonism she may feel towards him is the legacy of feelings which she had towards her parents, since he himself has not done anything to justify these feelings. If, however, she has had social contacts with him outside the consulting-room, he cannot always avoid remarks or actions which she will treat as, let us say, signs of hostility or affection, and in subsequent discussion in the consulting-room it may not be easy for him to decide—or to convince her—how little objective justification there was for her reactions. There is thus, by Freud's reasoning, a strong case for his rule against social contact with patients.

LENGTH OF TREATMENT

In the primitive phase, psychoanalysis had usually taken only a few weeks. Freud had confined himself to removing the hysterical symptoms which had led the patient to consult him. These presented themselves as physical symptoms, and he did not regard his technique as one for remedying disorders of the mind.[1] Consequently it is not surprising that he was able to regard his treatment as completed within such a short space of time. He soon began to realize, however, that his technique could be used to relieve symptoms that we should call mental, such as the unrealistic fears that are called 'phobias', or the need for some protective ritual that is called an 'obsession'. It was natural, too, that a technique which laid such stress on the development of the sexual feelings should be used in the treatment of sexual perversions. He was thus both raising his standards of 'cure' and taking on patients of types which, as we now know, respond much less quickly to psychotherapeutic treatment, and the result was that treatment became a much more lengthy affair. Patients now attended for an hour or two almost daily, and might do so for six months to three years.[2]

At the same time Freud had definite ideas about the limitations of his method. As early as 1904 he gave a list of the requirements which a patient must normally fulfil to be suitable for treatment:

(a) there must be periods during which she is 'psychically normal', so that he can communicate with her;

(b) she must have 'a certain measure of natural intelligence and ethical development' (this would, for example, exclude a moron and the conscienceless type known as a 'psychopath');

(c) she must not suffer from 'deep-rooted malformations of character, traits of an actually degenerate constitution', because these give rise to a 'resistance' that is almost impossible to overcome (it would have been interesting if he had been more specific here);

(d) she must be under fifty, for by then 'the mass of psychical material is no longer manageable . . . and the ability to undo psychical processes begins to grow weaker'.

It is a pity that he was not more specific under heading (c), for the rest of his list is surprisingly modern, and I do not think that many contemporary psychoanalysts would disagree with his

[1] In *Studies on Hysteria* (1895) he said, 'Much is won if we succeed in transforming hysterical misery into common unhappiness'.

[2] As Freud himself said in his anonymous article 'Freud's Psychoanalytic Procedure' (1904).

other three categories, although they might wish to add to their number.[1]

TRAINING OF PSYCHOANALYSTS

From about 1902 other doctors began to show an interest in Freud's methods, and to imitate them. Some relied merely on what they had heard or read. Those whose professional standards were higher—and they included Jung and Adler—learned from him by personal discussion. In 1907 Eitington, a Swiss doctor, underwent a short and informal psychoanalysis at Freud's hands out of pure interest in the procedure; this was the first training analysis. By 1910 Freud was becoming rather alarmed by the way in which people who had only imperfectly understood his methods were trying to practise them; the chief danger was that they would ascribe to every patient any peculiarities in their own personalities. In 1912 he therefore said very firmly that the only way to acquire the proper qualifications to practise psychoanalysis was to be psychoanalysed oneself. This has ever since been an invariable requirement of the Institutes which train psychoanalysts on orthodox lines in Europe and the United States. Freud himself never laid much stress on the advantages of a medical degree, but the desirability of 'lay psychoanalysts' has been fiercely debated since they began to appear in the nineteen-twenties in Europe and the United States. In Britain today a lay psychoanalyst who has undergone a prescribed training, including a lengthy psychoanalysis, is accepted by the British Psycho-Analytical Society only if he undertakes to accept no patients except those referred to him by medical practitioners, 'medical responsibility being retained in each case by a medical practitioner'. In the United States the official policy of the American Psychoanalytic Association and the institutes which it recognizes is opposed to the training of people without medical qualifications as psychoanalysts.[2]

---

[1] For example, although psychoanalytic methods are now used in some hospitals in the treatment of some psychoses, few psychoanalysts would claim that their normal technique is suitable for such disorders, unless in mild forms in young patients.

[2] *Practical and Theoretical Aspects of Psychoanalysis*, by L. Kubie, 1950.

B. Analysis of Ego and Transference

THEORETICAL DEVELOPMENTS

The third phase of psychoanalysis began about 1919, although it is possible to watch its incubation in Freud's writings from about 1912 onward. During the first world war his practice declined considerably,[1] and he was able to sit back and think about the theoretical implications of what he had been doing. In so far as this led to another improvement in his technique it was no doubt a fortunate breathing-space; but it also gave him the leisure to elaborate his explanatory model.

In some cases this was profitable. For example, he now emphasized a curious state of affairs that had been borne in upon him during the 'unconscious' phase. He had observed that under his technique his patients would confess to completely contradictory feelings—usually about their parents. A man who had, as a result of the technique, revived his strong childhood affection for his mother would in all probability at the same time revive an equally strong dislike of her; Freud called this 'ambivalence'. Another curious thing about the feelings which patients revealed was that they took no account of the passage of time. The fact that a man's father was dead, or old and feeble, did not prevent the man from fearing him as the omnipotent omniscient tyrant which he had appeared to be in the man's childhood. In this and other ways, the feelings and memories which the technique revived in patients did not behave in the same way as the thoughts of everyday conscious experience. Freud explained this by saying that the unconscious operated according to different laws, which he called collectively the 'primary process', since he thought that the rational, consistent, realistic way in which conscious thoughts were ordered was, from the evolutionary point of view, a later development. This is of course a technically valuable point, since it has an obvious moral for the psychoanalytic treatment of a patient. If under the technique the patient confesses to quite contradictory feelings towards the same object, neither feeling should be disregarded in subsequent analysis, and indeed until such contradictory feelings have

---

[1] Perhaps because the incidence of neurosis fell, as it did in Britain during the second world war. Another reason may have been that many of his patients had been drawn from other countries.

shown themselves there is a strong probability that the process of treatment has not been completed.

On the other hand, a good many of the ways in which Freud elaborated his model during this period were of very doubtful value technically. I have already mentioned his own qualms about the legitimacy of his notions of 'unfelt feelings', which arose from pedantic philosophical reasoning and were quite beside the point when dealing with a technical model. He managed, however, to evolve an explanation which satisfied him, and allowed him to continue, in effect, to use the idea of unconscious emotions, so that no harm was done. A more important development was his attempt to link up his introspective model, which consisted of desires, feelings, memories and all the other things that we can introspect, with the model of neurology. Neurology was his first love, and he had always cherished hopes of bridging the gap between mind and brain by describing the thoughts of the former in terms of the neurons and electric charges of the latter.[1] I have already mentioned how he visualized emotions as 'discharging' themselves when they became conscious. He now renewed this attempt, in what he called his 'metapsychology'. This attempted to describe not only the workings of the unconscious but also of the conscious mind in terms of Freud's nineteenth-century neurology. Concepts like 'reflex arcs',[2] 'cathexis', 'anti-cathexis', conscious, pre-conscious and unconscious 'systems', 'memory-traces', 'free' and 'bound' libido and so on, were pieced together into an elaborate theoretical apparatus, which from now on obtrudes itself constantly among the clear and interesting technical observations which Freud continued to make.

The problem with which Freud was faced was not of course an easy one. Although the entities of his model were copied from the phenomena of our introspectible minds, the model worked only if those entities were visualized as behaving somewhat differently. If this behaviour is very different from that of our conscious thoughts, is it worth retaining a model whose entities are copied from them? May this not be more misleading than helpful?

[1] About 1895 he attempted this in his 'Project D', but was apparently dissatisfied and never published it (it is now published in English translation, along with his letters to Fliess, under the title *The Origins of Psychoanalysis*, 1954).

[2] Taken from Wernicke's writings of the eighteen-seventies, and not from Pavlov, to whom Freud seems to have paid no attention.

It is important to remember at this point one peculiarity of psychotherapy as a technique. It has to deal with its material by talking to it. This means that its terminology must not only be helpful to the technician himself in thinking about his material; it must also be such as to influence his material in the way he wants to. In other words, the most precise and elaborate model has no influence on the patient if she cannot understand it. There is no doubt that the patient must co-operate in the treatment if it is to succeed; and that if she is to co-operate she must have an idea of what the technician is trying to do. One of the virtues of the model of unconscious memories and feelings is that it can be easily understood by patients. Indeed, I think that it has a positive suggestive value. There is a laboratory experiment called the 'body-sway test of suggestibility', in which the subject stands blind-folded while a voice says to him 'You are falling forward . . . You are falling forward . . .' As a result, most subjects do sway forward to a greater or lesser extent. I have already pointed out how the model of unconscious feelings enabled Freud to think of the feelings of childhood as still present in the patient, and therefore still capable of being manipulated, instead of being inaccessible in the distant past; this is the diagnostic use of the model. But I think that it also enabled him to make the patient think of these feelings as still present, and thus have the confidence that they could be revived. If the experimenter merely said 'You used to fall when you were a child, and you *could* fall forward now if you tried' his results would be far less spectacular. In the same way the psycho-analyst's attempts to revive his patient's childhood feelings would, I think, be less effective if instead of describing them to his patient as still present in her unconscious, he could only talk of them as in the past. This is the suggestive use of the model of the unconscious.

What Freud seems to have decided is that while he must continue to use this model in talking to his patients he would have to use a more complicated one in thinking about them; he would have one model for diagnostic purposes and retain the old one for suggestive purposes. This may or may not have been the right decision; we shall see how later psychotherapeutic schools tried to meet this undoubted difficulty. Where he did, I think, make a mistake was in trying to use a neurological model for diagnostic purposes. In the first place, his neurology was out-of-date. In the second place, not even present-day neurology is able to provide a model that is useful in psychotherapeutic techniques. The model of present-day neurology is useful in some non-semantic techniques—for example, in severing connections between the frontal lobes and the rest of the brain, in passing electrical currents through the cortex, or in locating damage by electro-encephalography. But the very complexity of the structure of the brain and its relationship to the other systems of our bodies which are involved in emotional disorders means that the neurological model is far too complicated for the man of average intellect to grasp, let alone use in working out what he must say to a patient who is being treated semantically.

Freud's metapsychology is therefore a pseudo-neurological model, and it is one of the unfortunate and slightly dangerous things about modern orthodox psychoanalysis that it has continued to use it. It is dangerous because it can mislead its users into thinking that they are using a corresponding model, which is therefore likely to have universal validity and which is unlikely to need the constant revision that technical models ought to have. It may even mislead them into using the model to work out what must be the cause, and then clinging to this idea, instead of using the only safe test, which is to see whether this assumption cures the patient.

THE 'EGO' AND THE 'ID'

One theoretical change, however, was of such importance from the technical point of view that it can be regarded as the beginning of the modern phase of orthodox psychoanalysis. Freud had been paying more and more attention to the way in which his patients used to resist his efforts to help them in the process of anamnesis. This phenomenon, which he called 'resistance', was quite involuntary, and was very difficult to overcome, even by drawing patients' attention to the way in which they were thus delaying their own recovery. Freud had at first explained this by saying that the repressed memories and feelings had been repressed because they were repugnant to consciousness; but now he began to ask himself why they were repugnant. He no longer took it for granted that such thoughts are repressed, but wondered why our consciousness is so constituted that it does repress them. In order to explain this he had to think of it in rather a different way. Instead of visualizing it simply as a region of the mind, which thoughts entered and left, he began to think of it as an organization of thoughts with a character of its own, which insisted on having a say in the question of which thoughts should be allowed to enter. It was no longer a mere hotel, which any thought could use so long as there was room, but a club, whose members could blackball or expel unwanted entrants. This club he called the 'ego', and the rest of the mind, consisting of the instinctual desires and the repressed emotional experiences, he named the 'id'.[1]

Part of the ego's organization specializes in deciding which thoughts should be allowed membership of it. This part, which Freud called the 'super-ego' (Uberich) because of its dominance over the rest of the ego, is not inborn, but is the result of parental influence. At first the child consciously refrains from doing something 'because Daddy wouldn't like it'. If the prohibition or the temptation is very strong, the child may find it easier not even to think of doing it, since thinking is very close to doing (particularly with young children). In later life the child may occasionally consider a course of action quite consciously in the light of what its parents would have approved; but its chronic acts of repression will be sustained quite automatically, so that it will not be conscious of the operation of this part of the ego. It is as if the club had suffered in its early days from some rather badly behaved members, to whom its attention had been drawn once or twice by the authorities. After one or two expulsions it found itself with a small unofficial committee which scrutinized applications for membership. As time went on they did their work more and more smoothly and unobtrusively, although occasionally, when a rather unusual application was received, they had to call an official meeting. Sometimes one of the rejected applicants got past their scrutiny by assuming a heavy disguise, and at night when the committee were not there, some of the undesirables would come in and misbehave in the club's premises. But on the whole they kept the club respectable.

[1] Freud's own terms were 'Ich' and 'es', but in English they are always translated thus. The ego was derived, in conception if not in name, from Herbart and Nietzsche, the id from Groddeck (see Appendix B). The first incorporation of this distinction in Freud's writings was in *The Ego and the Id*, published in 1923; but the concept of the ego had been incubating in his mind for some years.

DEFENCE-MECHANISMS

By 1926 Freud had also changed his views on the subject of repression. Hitherto he had regarded this as the only way in which the conscious ego could deal with an experience that was too repugnant to be borne. Now he distinguished several ways in which the ego defended itself. He was now seventy years of age, and the detailed study and classification of what have come to be called the 'defence-mechanisms' was carried on by his successors, notably his daughter, Anna Freud, and Wilhelm Reich. It is striking how the history of psychoanalysis proper from 1896 to 1926 is largely the intellectual biography of one man. There were of course the apostasies of Adler and Jung, which I shall be considering in the next three chapters; and there were minor additions to theory which I have not considered worth the room they would occupy. But the developments that were of real technical importance were the work of Freud himself. Nor did he cease to play an active part in further developments even at the age of seventy; his last book —an extremely clear exposition of his theory in popular terms— was begun in 1938, only a short time before his death at the age of eighty-four. From 1926 onward, however, the major developments, even in orthodox psychoanalysis, were the work of others.

Freud pointed out that in addition to repression there were the following defence-mechanisms:

Regression: the relapsing into an earlier stage of instinctual gratification (such as the oral stage) because of some obstacle to the proper development of a more mature stage (such as the genital).

Sublimation: the direction of the energy of an unacceptable instinct (such as the sexual) into more acceptable channels (such as portrait painting).

Projection: the ascribing to someone else of feelings or motives that one dare not admit in oneself.

Isolation: the refusal to see a particular way of thinking or behaving in its relationship to the rest of one's thoughts or behaviour (as, for example, child-beating and blood-sports are taught at Christian schools).

Other psychoanalysts have added to this list. Ernest Jones had already drawn attention, for example, to

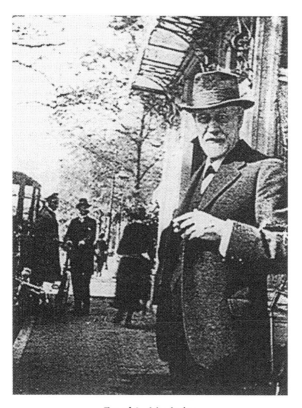

Freud in his sixties.

[to face page 50

Rationalization: the manufacturing of a respectable conscious motive for thoughts or actions really prompted by disreputable, repressed desires. (For example, 'I only smoke because it makes me better-tempered.')

The technical innovation which accompanied this development in theory was the paying of more attention, in treatment, to the patient's reasons for repressing or otherwise defending herself against her unconscious. It was still necessary to aim at the anamnesis of repressed experiences, but this was done chiefly in order to make conscious not only the parental influence that has made the patient feel guilty about these experiences, but also the exact way in which the patient had disposed of them. This innovation was at first known as 'analysing the resistance' but is now generally called 'ego-analysis': it was, of course, an innovation in topic rather than a new intermediate technique.

TRANSFERENCE

It was natural that these developments should be accompanied by increasing attention to the phenomenon of transference, that striking mixture of affection and dislike which the patient manifests towards the psychoanalyst in the course of treatment. At first, as we have seen, Freud regarded it as an unavoidable nuisance. Later he came to see that he could use the patient's dependence on him to overcome her resistance; if she wanted to please him she should co-operate in the process of reviving the past. Finally, he recognized the very close resemblance between the phenomenon of transference and the patient's childhood feelings towards her own parents. His followers, particularly in England, began to use 'analysis of the transference' as a special kind of ego-analysis. The patient's feelings towards the analyst would be dragged into consciousness, discussed and interpreted as revivals of her attitude towards her parents in infancy. By the time Freud died, it was being suggested that the analysis of the transference was as important as the revival of the past in curing the patient.

So far in this short historical account I have ignored not only minor points of theory (particularly where they seemed to me to have no practical bearing on technique) but also the minor and major divergences from Freud's theory and technique which were introduced from time to time after 1910. I shall try to deal in the following chapters with the major divergences, including the main variants that have survived, or arose during, the last war; for the minor ones there is not space. I have, however, tried to include in this outline all the important technical developments in the main stream of Freudian psychoanalysis, and this seems a good point at which to summarize its main features.

ORTHODOX PSYCHOANALYSIS

In the hands of Freud himself[1] and of his orthodox followers psychoanalysis is a psychotherapeutic sub-technique which aims at the cure or alleviation of certain psychic and somatic symptoms by two intermediate techniques. These are

(i) the anamnesis of the patient's childhood experiences and phantasies, with particular attention to the topic of sexuality;
(ii) the interpretation of the patient's present unconscious feelings, with particular attention to the topics of
   (*a*) transference
   (*b*) the defence-mechanisms of the ego.

In both intermediate techniques, but particularly in anamnesis, free association is used as a facilitant, but not hypnosis or drugs. Orthodox Freudians do not consider that the sub-technique can be properly applied by those who have not undergone a thorough training, including a personal analysis. It is not often used in treating

the elderly;
adults with marked hallucinations, delusions or other forms of dissociation from reality;
adults or adolescents of the type (sometimes called 'psychopaths') who seem to lack a moral sense;
adults, adolescents or children whose intelligence is too low for an easy exchange of thoughts.

[1] Some people, who sought analysis from Freud towards the end of his life—in several cases out of curiosity, professional or ordinary—have given reports of his methods which suggest that he broke all his own rules: see, for example, Helen W. Puner's biography of Freud. But this does not mean that he broke them when he was dealing with genuinely ill patients in his middle age. After all, 'old men forget'.

It very seldom takes less than six months, and usually stretches over several years; it is usually conducted in sessions of 45 to 60 minutes, once a day on two to five days a week. The patient usually lies on a couch, with the psychoanalyst out of sight. During treatment the psychoanalyst tries to avoid giving her advice on the conduct of her everyday life, and to confine his intervention strictly to the content of treatment; and he also avoids any social contact outside the consulting-room.

In communicating with patients he uses an introspective model of unconscious thoughts which is modelled on the conscious phenomena studied by introspection; onto this has been grafted the model of an ego which defends itself at the instruction of a superego from unwelcome thoughts. In technical discussion amongst themselves, however, psychoanalysts tend to use terms which imply a pseudo-neurological model drawn from Freud's nineteenth-century neurological researches.

It has several other implications and assumptions which seem to me to be of importance, particularly when it is compared with other sub-techniques.

In the first place it is *deterministic*. It looks for a cause for every human change in the present state—mental or physical—of that human being. The idea of a person being drawn onward by a goal, a 'final cause', is foreign to it, except in so far as that goal is represented in the person's present state by a conscious or unconscious thought of that goal.

Its implications, however, are not as *materialistic* as the Edwardian Christians feared. Freud himself did not believe that mind and body were two separate substances; he saw them in much the same way as that other great Jew, Spinoza—both seemed to be aspects of the same substance, each acting according to laws that belonged to their spheres, but having the unconscious as a sort of interpreter between them. Unlike techniques that relieve mental symptoms by physical interference with the brain, psychoanalysis can be regarded by dualists as operating through the mind in just the same way as moral exhortations do. Where it does conflict with traditional Christianity is in seeing moral judgments not as the effect of an intuition through which an eternal truth is revealed but as the legacy of parental influence before the age of six. But theologians and moral philosophers have, in time, reconciled wider differences than this.

It is also what I call *'egalitarian'*, in the sense that it pays as little attention as possible to hereditary differences between one person and another. Just as in the seventeenth century Locke regarded the mind of the new-born child as a clean sheet (*'tabula rasa'*) on which all its ideas were inscribed by its subsequent experience, so psychoanalysis treats the psychological differences between human beings as acquired and not inherited. It is true that in the early phases Freud talked about an inherited disposition towards neurosis, and even in his later years recognized that the strength of a particular instinct in one man might be greater than in another. But his technique concentrates on the psychological peculiarities that are acquired in the individual's history. It regards any peculiarities that it does succeed in treating as being acquired characteristics, and so reduces to the minimum the portion of the individual's personality which is attributed to inheritance.

It is also what I call *'optimistic'*. I do not merely mean that it assumes, unless it can be convinced of the contrary, that psychological abnormality is acquired and therefore curable; I also mean that, within the field in which it claims to be effective, its approach implies a belief in what the old physicians used to call the *'vis medicatrix naturae'*,—the healing power of nature. If a wound in an otherwise healthy person is kept clean, more or less closed, and protected from interference, it will heal. In much the same way many psychoanalysts assume that if the childhood tangle of feelings and prohibitions can be brought into the light of consciousness it will straighten itself out without active interference. Indeed, they believe that better and more permanent results are achieved in this way than by more active intervention.

Recommended Reading
(*in addition to that recommended in Chapter II*)

PSYCHOANALYSIS: EVOLUTION AND DEVELOPMENT, by Clara Thompson. Allen and Unwin, 1952.

AN OUTLINE OF PSYCHOANALYSIS, by Sigmund Freud, tr. J. Strachey. W. W. Norton, 1949.

IV

INDIVIDUAL PSYCHOLOGY AND COUNSELLING

ALFRED ADLER (1870–1937) was born and educated in Vienna. Like Freud he was a Jew. It is probably significant in the light of his theories that he was a delicate child, who suffered from rickets and a violent spasm of the glottis; he also seems to have been what we should nowadays call 'accident-prone'. He qualified as a physician in 1895 and after a year or two in the Viennese Hospital and Policlinic became an eye-specialist for a short time; this was followed by a year or two of general practice, after which he was encouraged by Kraft-Ebing's lectures to take up neurology. It was during this period that he married Raissa Epstein, a Russian who was an intimate friend of Trotsky; he himself, and many of his immediate followers, were enthusiastic socialists. In 1902, after a lecture by Freud to the Viennese Society of Medicine had aroused his interest in psychoanalysis, he was invited by Freud to join a discussion-group, of which the other original members were Stekel, Kahane and Reitler; in 1910 Freud, who had a considerable affection for him, made him President of what had now grown into a small society, and together with Stekel he became editor of the *Zentralblatt für Psychoanalyse*. By this time, however, he had begun to disagree openly with Freud on several important points, and in 1911 he resigned from the Society and (at Freud's request) from the co-editorship of the *Zentralblatt*, to found a small group of his own. This was at first given the pointed title of 'Society for Free Psychoanalysis', but in 1912 was renamed 'The Society for Individual Psychology'.

Long before this final breach, however, Adler had begun to develop ideas of his own. In 1907 he had published a book called *Studies of Organ Inferiority*, in which he had drawn attention to

55

some interesting facts about defective bodily organs. In the first place, he pointed out how often a tendency to some defect of a particular organ occurs in more than one member of the same family; he instanced a family in which the grandfather died from tuberculosis of the kidney, the father suffered from stones in the bladder, one of his children had cancer of the kidney and another was a bed-wetter. Moreover, one individual could have a susceptibility to afflictions of one particular organ. Some patients, for example, seem to specialize in disorders of the digestive tract, others in disease of the respiratory system. His next observation was that when this happens the body often develops in such a way as to compensate for the defect. If one kidney is defective, the other grows large enough to do the work of both; and unpaired organs, such as the heart, may become larger than normal in order to counterbalance a defect which prevents them from being fully efficient in their normal state. This compensation could even reach a level at which it overdid matters and became 'over-compensation'. He went on to observe that in addition to this purely somatic kind of compensation there was a psychic compensation. A child with congenital word-blindness which made it very difficult to read written symbols, such as words or numbers, not only managed to overcome this defect but actually became an accountant. History is full of other examples; Demosthenes' stammer, Beethoven's deafness, F. S. Smythe's weak heart.

These observations of what he called 'organ-inferiority' suggested to Adler that the abnormal symptoms of neurotics could be explained in a somewhat similar way. In their case it was seldom possible to point to any particular defective organ and to say that their consciousness of its defectiveness had determined their behaviour; but it was, he thought, possible to explain their behaviour by assuming a general sense of inferiority—the 'inferiority complex'. A boy, for example, who has an elder brother will often be very conscious of his brother's superior strength and skill, and will probably try very hard to equal or surpass him, either by practising hard the things the brother does well or by cultivating some accomplishment at which the brother is not so outstanding. Adler himself was the second of six children, got on very badly with his elder brother, and always emphasized the effect of a child's place in the sequence of birth upon its character and behaviour. Such behaviour is not always, of course, neurotic. But some children, who are unable to gain their goal of superiority by direct competition, find that if they are ill they can achieve attention, privileges and thus superiority of a kind. This discovery leads them to withdraw from the healthy competition and other demands of communal life and take refuge in illness, physical or mental,[1] whose form is determined partly by their inherited constitution, partly by the accidents of early life. Thus there is formed what Adler calls the 'life-style'[2] of the individual, which determines the course of the remainder of his life.

Because of the accepted superiority of men, women suffered from the inferiority complex in a particularly intense form. Since men are dominant, women must want to be men. This 'masculine protest', as Adler called it, explains not only those women who are obviously trying to be more male than a man, or the dominant partners in Lesbian relationships, but also, in a less obvious way, women who prefer a succession of love-affairs to settling down as the subordinate partner of one man. Frigidity was explained as the refusal to submit to male domination, and prostitutes (who are often frigid) were really intent on degrading men to the level of mere means of subsistence. The masculine protest is of course intensified if in childhood the girl realizes that her parents would have wished her to be a boy.

THE FUNDAMENTAL FORCES

Adler thus regarded all forms of faulty development as due to various manifestations of the drive for domination, the will-to-power.[3] Normal development of personality, on the other hand, took place under the influence of what he called the 'community-feeling'. This is 'eternal, real and physiologically rooted' and out of it are developed 'tenderness, love of neighbour, friendship and

---

[1] The notion of 'gain from illness' is found in a paper published by Freud in 1909, to which Adler probably owed it.

[2] Sometimes called the 'life-line' or 'life-pattern'.

[3] Rudolf Dreikurs points out in *Present Day Psychology* (ed. A. A. Roback), 1955, that in his last works, which were based on his popular lectures, Adler modified the will-to-power into a drive to overcome obstacles. Had he lived longer it would have been interesting to see whether this would have led to important modifications in his theory or technique; as it is, he may merely have been presenting the will-to-power in a more favourable light, without really altering his views on the part it played in disorder.

love'. We have seen how Freud regarded the development of personality as due to the interaction between two psychic forces — the pleasure-seeking libido and the destructive instinct of aggression (a notion which probably owed something to Adler's influence). Adler seems to have felt the same need for two interacting forces, and arrived at the notions of the will-to-power and the community-feeling. As I have said, he and many of his immediate circle were enthusiastic socialists, and there can be no doubt that the notion of the community-feeling as a fundamental psychic force was derived from the socialist's faith in man's future as a political animal. What is slightly less obvious is that the notion of the will-to-power as the vitiating force in human development is also due to Adler's socialism. Domination by an individual was just as abhorrent to nineteenth-century socialism as it was to the democratic Greeks and republican Romans of the pre-Christian era, or to the Frenchmen of the revolutionary period. Since Adler believed that man at his best was a socialist comrade, it was natural that he should regard man at his worst as a would-be dictator.

There is, however, a very important difference between the Freudian and the Adlerian explanation of neurotic symptoms. Freud saw them as the result of conflict between two groups of irreconcilable instincts. While Adler also believed in two kinds of instinct, he regarded healthy or neurotic behaviour as produced not by interaction between them but by one or other of them, whichever had ascendancy in that particular person. This enabled him to claim that his system treated the person as an undivided whole, whose thoughts and feelings could be understood only by grasping the goal at which the entire organism was aiming; hence the name 'individual psychology', which meant 'the psychology of the indivisible personality'.

TECHNIQUE

Unlike most of Freud's circle Adler was never analysed by Freud; what he learned of psychoanalytic technique was gleaned from the weekly discussions and the reading of papers by the Freudians, and not from practical experience of it. The method which he developed had therefore several features in common with Freud's, but owed more to Adler's own personality and ideas.

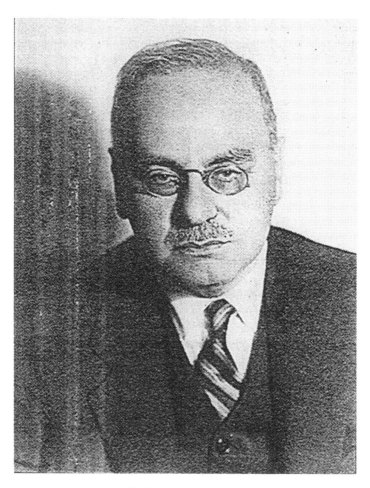

Alfred Adler in his sixties.

[to face page 58

Unlike Freud, Adler was a forceful, energetic, impatient man, with an exceptional capacity for converting other people—and particularly large audiences—to his point of view by his clear and attractive manner of speaking. He wanted, and was often able to get, quick results with his neurotic patients. He was also unlike Freud in having no early experience of hypnotism and its derivative techniques to make him fear that he might be using suggestion. The essence of his technique therefore consisted in convincing the patient by the evidence of her own behaviour that she was using her symptoms as means to achieve the particular kind of power over others which she had chosen as her goal. His own description of the process is interesting:

> . . . *the uncovering of the neurotic life-plan* proceeds apace in friendly and free conversation, it being always the *better tactics to let the patient take the initiative.* I found it the safest course to search for and merely unmask the neurotic line of operation as shown in expression and in the train of thought, and at the same time thus unobtrusively educate the patient for the same kind of work. The physician must be so convinced of the *uniqueness and exclusiveness of the neurotic direction-line* that he is able to call up the true content [of the patient's mind], always telling him beforehand his disturbing 'arrangements' and constructions, and trying to discover and explain until the patient, completely upset, gives them up in order to place new and better hidden ones in their place. How often this will occur it is impossible to say beforehand. Finally, however, the patient will give in, all the more easily, if his relation to the physician has not permitted the feeling of a [possible] defeat to develop.[1]

INTERPRETATION

Adler's chief intermediate technique is thus interpretation, which plays an even more important part in his treatment than in Freud's. Indeed, where Freud would try by free association to induce the patient to be the first to put his desires and feelings into words and would use interpretation only where this failed, Adler would not hesitate to interpret to the patient what she was doing

[1] *Individual Psychology*, 1913.

as soon as *he* saw it clearly, without waiting until *she* did. The material which he interpreted was of four main kinds:

(1) *The patient's behaviour and conscious thoughts inside and outside the consulting-room.* A man's choice of a career, for example, and his relationships with women were seen either as fulfilments of his unconscious desire for domination or compensations for some unconsciously felt inferiority. His reactions to treatment and attitude to the psychotherapist were interpreted along the same lines, as we shall see when considering Adler's use of the transference.

(2) *The patient's symptoms.* Adler often saw in the form which her symptoms took a symbol of her unconscious feelings. A sufferer from giddiness and fears of falling was probably afraid of a moral lapse. Writer's cramp was attributed to dislike of a task or job which involved writing.

(3) *The patient's dreams.* Like Freud, he saw the dream as a distorted reflection of unconscious wishes; but whereas Freud saw them as disguised fulfilments of those wishes, Adler saw them as attempts to suggest a way of achieving the dreamer's life-plan. We shall see later that Jung also saw a purposive element in dreams.

(4) *The patient's earliest memories.* These seemed to him to be important, but only as clues to the way in which the patient's life-plan had been determined. He asked over a hundred doctors for their first childhood memory, and found that in most cases it was of a serious illness or the death of some member of their family.

ANAMNESIS

Freud, as we have seen, paid great attention to the recovery of early memories because he believed in the cathartic value of this process. Adler, on the other hand, laid so much emphasis on interpretation that, as we have just seen, he used early memories solely as material for interpretation. What was more, the whole point of an early memory for him was that it was accessible without the use of special sub-techniques; he was interested in the reason why the patient remembered this incident and not others. He therefore took no special steps to revive lost memories.

TRANSFERENCE

Although Adler seems to have had an extraordinary capacity for attracting and converting people of all ages and sexes, his relationship with his patients was coloured by what he saw as the struggle for domination. Since his aim was, crudely speaking, to detect and expose the neurotic stratagems of his patients as quickly as possible, it is not surprising that their antagonism was aroused; and of course his insistence on interpreting all their behaviour in terms of the aggressive striving for superiority no doubt encouraged this reaction. However this may be, his patients seemed to him to be fighting against the inferior position in which the relationship placed them. Any friendship which he was able to establish he saw not as a manifestation of the child's affection for a quasi-parental figure but as a vestige of the group-consciousness which had been obliterated by the neurosis.

RE-EDUCATION

While Freud took pains not to give his patients any positive injunctions as to their future way of life, and saw himself merely as the midwife who brought out what was in them, Adler had very definite views about the principles which ought to govern the conduct of the cured neurotic. His socialism convinced him that the proper function of man was participation in and service to the life of the community; any kind of withdrawal from this was an unhealthy symptom; 'to cure a neurosis and a psychosis it is necessary to change completely the whole upbringing of the patient and turn him definitely and unconditionally back upon society'.[1] We should, I think, be justified in regarding what Adler called 're-education' as a separate intermediate technique, which was Adler's addition to those evolved by Freud.

SEXUALITY

Although Freud abandoned at quite an early stage his theory that neurotic symptoms had their origin in incidents that were literally sexual, he not only regarded the pleasure derived from all pleasurable behaviour as being of the same sensual kind, which he

---

[1] *Individual Psychology*, 1913.

called erotic, but also continued to attach great importance to the full investigation of his patients' sexual behaviour in the narrow sense. It was of course this feature of his theory and technique that made them so controversial, and there is no doubt that one of the reasons why Adler's theories were welcomed was that they laid so little emphasis on sexuality that they could be discussed in any drawing-room. The question whether all pleasure should be regarded as sexual in nature is very largely a theoretical or even metaphysical one; but the extent to which a psychotherapist insists that his patient should talk about her sexual feelings and behaviour is of course a most important point of technique. Adler did not of course avoid the discussion of sexual matters, particularly if the patient seemed to want this or if the symptoms of which she complained were obviously sexual. Even so, however, he regarded sexual behaviour as merely one manifestation of the patient's striving for domination, and any sexual abnormalities were interpreted by him in this way.[1]

THE ADLERIAN UNCONSCIOUS

But Adler's 'individual' or, as we should call it, unitary approach to personality, which dispensed with the notion of conflict within the person, led to a much more important divergence from Freud which he made without fully appreciating it. Adler's technique consisted, broadly speaking, of inducing his patients to recognize the goal which they were trying to achieve and to recognize how their symptoms were calculated to achieve it. Freud's consisted of inducing them to feel emotions and desires which they were refusing to feel. There is a very great difference between recognizing a fact about oneself and feeling an emotion; I may be afraid of someone and yet unwilling to recognize that I am afraid. Most middle-aged men are unwilling to admit that they are still afraid of their old headmasters, but when they meet them experience a feeling which, whatever they call it, is fear. Some men, however, are so determined not to feel fear that in the same circumstances they are able to subdue this feeling (although they may of course exhibit other symptoms, such as restlessness or a dry mouth). The

[1] It is very difficult to explain by means of Adler's theories how a woman can ever find the female sexual role completely satisfactory; and I cannot find any passage in which he really faces this problem.

first kind of men are refusing to recognize a fact about themselves, while the second are refusing to feel an emotion. Freud's technique was aimed at overcoming the refusal to feel emotions when this took the exaggerated and chronic form which he called repression. Adler's technique, on the other hand, had the effect of inducing his patients to recognize unpalatable facts about themselves, and to recognize how their symptoms fitted in with those facts. For Adler, although he did not clearly appreciate this, repression is merely failure to recognize. As a result, the Adlerian description of the unconscious is a catalogue of facts which the patient will not admit— such as her struggle to dominate her family; while the Freudian description is a catalogue of emotions and desires which the patient refuses to feel—such as hate for her parents. As time went on Adler used the word 'unconscious' less and less frequently, and even said 'the use of the terms "consciousness" and "unconsciousness" to designate distinctive mental factors is incorrect in the practice of Individual Psychology'.[1]

THE 'CASUAL' VERSUS THE 'PURPOSIVE' APPROACH

Adler also emphasized that whereas Freud explained thoughts and actions as the effect of past events, individual psychology did so in terms of the future events which were their goals. In this he was followed by Jung. They condemned psychoanalysis as a 'causal' approach; in their view it explained and treated neurosis entirely by reference to what had gone wrong, as if the patient were a mere mechanism, whereas her symptoms could be fully understood only if they were seen as an attempt to deal with her difficulties. At first sight this looks like another version of the Aristotelian doctrine of 'final causes' and the attempt to regard living matter as subject to causation of a metaphysically different sort, against which scientists have fought a successful battle in the last century or two. Certainly Freud's explanation is of the sort which science has tried to provide for all kinds of phenomena, organic and inorganic. Freudians would no doubt argue, too, that the 'goals' of Adler and Jung influence our behaviour only because they are represented in us by a conception of them and a desire for them, however vague or unconscious these may be; if so, they are 'causes' of the ordinary antecedent sort, and not merely future possibilities.

[1] *The Science of Living*, 1929.

In order to argue effectively on these lines they have of course to make considerable use of the Freudian model of unconscious mental events, and the Adlerian and Jungian viewpoint is thus connected with the much more superficial use which their theories make of this model.[1] What is more, Jungians and Adlerians might point out that even the Freudian notion of an instinct involves the concept of a goal, since the only way, for example, in which it is possible to explain the difference between the sexual and the aggressive instincts is by reference to their aims, which are pleasure and destruction.

The modern logician tends to take the view that the two kinds of explanation are not necessarily incompatible, and that the 'purposive' type may simply be the only one possible in a particular field until we have acquired a certain degree of precision in our formulation of 'causal' laws.[2] But in this particular instance of the controversy, we are, I think, faced with one more example of the importance of remembering that we are dealing not with a science but with a technique. From the point of view of the psychotherapists, the important question is whether better results are achieved by reviving past experiences and making conscious the present conflicts or by discussing with the patient what she might do in the future. As we have seen, Freudians are at great pains to avoid not only suggestion but also positive advice to the patient on the conduct of her life outside the consulting-room; whereas Adler introduced the intermediate technique of 're-education', which was adopted, although in a more subtle form, by Jung. Indeed, both Adler and Jung might be described as having searched in their patients for traces of desirable tendencies (in Adler's case the social as opposed to the anti-social tendencies) which they proceeded to encourage.

ADLERIAN PSYCHOTHERAPY

The sub-technique developed by Adler is thus one which makes little use of anamnesis, but a more active use of interpretation than psychoanalysis, and which employs one intermediate technique— re-education—that is deliberately avoided by orthodox psycho-

[1] I am of course thinking only of the 'personal unconscious', and disregarding, for the moment, Jung's notion of the 'collective unconscious'.
[2] See, for example, *Scientific Explanation*, by R. B. Braithwaite, 1946.

analysis. As the main topics for interpretation and re-education it selects the will-to-power, inferiority feelings and the community-feeling. Its explanatory model is a much simpler and more superficial form of the Freudian unconscious. Like psychoanalysis it employs regular sessions of 45 to 60 minutes, but is usually content with about two sessions a week, whereas some Freudians, as we have seen, aim at five a week. The Adlerian sees no particular reason to avoid social intercourse with his patient. The period of treatment is usually much shorter than in psychoanalysis, but Freudians would claim that this is because it is less thorough, and may leave untreated the fundamental causes of neuroses. Men and women without medical qualifications are accepted as members of the Societies of Individual Psychologists in the U.S.A. and by the Adlerian Society of Great Britain; but the Alfred Adler Medical Society in Britain admits only medical practitioners. All these groups consider a personal analysis desirable as part of training, but none appear to insist on it.

What distinguished Adler's fundamental approach most plainly from that of Freud was a tendency to import moral judgments into his attitude towards his patients, a tendency which is still to be seen in some individual psychologists. The patient is in his view not so much the victim of circumstances as a person who has made the wrong choice of a way of life at an earlier stage, and who must be made to see that it was and is wrong; the right choice is always the social one. This attitude is of course closely connected with the intermediate technique of re-education; a re-educator is very likely to have his own ideas as to what his patient should be like, and if so can hardly avoid forcing them upon her. We shall see, however, when we come to Jung's technique that this *a priori* approach is not essential to this intermediate technique.

AFTER ADLER

The Adlerian point of view survives in two forms. In the first place, there are psychotherapists who deliberately label themselves 'individual psychologists'. Most of these belong to small groups in such European capitals as Vienna, Paris, Amsterdam and London, and in New York, Chicago and Los Angeles in the United States, where there are training institutes and child guidance centres run on Adler's principles. There is also an International Association of Individual Psychology. There have been slight changes in the emphasis laid on Adler's intermediate techniques. The transference, for instance, has come to be seen as a means of ensuring the patient's co-operation in treatment, and more attention is therefore paid to the establishment of a good relationship between patient and psychotherapist. This use of the transference as a facilitant rather than a topic for interpretation was, as we have seen, a stage through which Freudian psychoanalysis passed. But no new intermediate techniques or topics have been introduced, and in consequence there have been no major modifications of theory.

Adler's importance seems to me, however, to lie mainly in his influence on other schools of psychotherapy. It is very likely, for example, that his notion of the will-to-power led Freud to substitute aggression for self-preservation as the second fundamental instinct, which opposed the libido. We shall see, too, how his intermediate technique of re-education has been adopted, wittingly or unwittingly, by Jung, and how the latter in consequence resembles Adler in emphasizing the 'purposive' view of neurosis as distinct from the 'causal' view of the Freudians. It is probably in the U.S.A., however, that his influence has been strongest. Not only do the 'cultural' group of neo-Freudians resemble him in their attention to the patient's present attitude towards other people, and their comparative neglect of childhood memories, but there is also a tendency to use an Adlerian model of the basic human drives, which we shall see in the approach of Rogers. Adler's explicit watering-down of the notion of the unconscious is also reflected in Rogers' avoidance of the term. His contribution to the development of group psychotherapy was probably not so great as that of followers of his, such as Rudolf Dreikurs and Joshua Bierer (see Chapter IX).

Counselling

In the United States between the wars an increasing number of child guidance clinics employed workers—with a wide variety of qualifications—to advise parents on the upbringing and careers of their children. Universities and similar establishments also began to employ men and women who specialized in advising students not only on the sort of vocations that were suited to their capabilities but also, as time went on, about more personal problems. The technique of 'counselling' thus grew up in a number of scattered places, without any one person as its father and consequently without any one theory as its basis (although every practitioner must have had his own preconceptions). This orphan-like childhood makes it almost unique among psychotherapeutic sub-techniques, and may not have been a complete misfortune. One important consequence was that its methods were shaped very much by the nature of the patients (or 'clients', as counsellors call them) who presented themselves. In the child guidance clinics these were of course parents who felt the need of positive advice about the handling of their children; while in the Universities they were adolescent boys and girls who had not yet outgrown their dependence on adults for advice and control. The result was that the counsellors were expected to tell these parents or adolescents what to do, not only in such practical matters as bed-time for infants or the right career for a boy with mathematical ability, but even in such emotional problems as shyness, unpopularity or inability to study. Many of the problems with which they had to deal were not of course psychotherapeutic ones, but to those that were their approach was inevitably that of the authoritative advisor. In many cases their methods were undoubtedly 'suggestive' (see Chapter VIII).

In dealing, however, with neurosis there is a very decided limit to the effectiveness either of suggestion or of direction. Someone, for example, who is afraid of going out of doors unaccompanied can be told that this fear will gradually disappear as he gets older; or he can be shown how to order his life so as to minimize the effects of this handicap. Between them these measures may make his life more tolerable; but it is unlikely that this is his only symptom or that it will disappear permanently or completely as a result of such suggestions. Gradually therefore the counsellors came under the influence of psychoanalytic ways of thinking. The chief agent of this influence was Carl Rogers (1902–), who after working in the New York Institute of Child Guidance became Director of the Rochester Guidance Center and subsequently Professor of Psychology at Chicago University.

In the nineteen-thirties Rogers advocated the use of the 'personality-testing' techniques evolved in the laboratories; on these he based a diagnosis of the patient, as a result of which he gave certain advice. Gradually, however, his experience led him to attach less importance to 'diagnosis' and 'direction', and more to the relationship between the 'counsellor' and his 'client', and his technique clearly came under the influence of the Freudians and Adlerians. Nevertheless, one of the striking things about his writings is the extent to which he avoids their technical terms. The most obvious example of this is where he is talking of feelings which the Freudian or Adlerian would describe as 'unconscious' or 'repressed'; Rogers prefers to refer to them as 'unexpressed' or as 'not yet brought into full consciousness'. He also gives a very clear description of the phenomenon which Freudians and Jungians call 'transference'—that alternation in the patient of dislike and affection for the psychotherapist; but he simply describes it as 'positive or negative feelings towards the counsellor'. Another way in which he differs from Freudians, Adlerians and Jungians is in offering no theory about man's basic drives and motivations. He makes no suggestion that patients are motivated by any impulses other than those which are familiar to consciousness; although some people are less able than others to recognize and accept these impulses. It is noticeable, however, that a very large proportion of his patients' recorded conversations, and of the counsellor's interpretations, deal with the idea of 'hostility', and it may well be as a result of Adler's influence that he pays so much attention to this motive.

He does, however, have a very definite theory about the nature of the curative factor in counselling. In his view the patient improves partly through catharsis—through the 'release of expression', partly through 'insight', and partly through the assistance given to a natural potentiality for recovery. We have seen that when Freud relied entirely on anamnesis he too believed that catharsis was the secret of his technique, but that when he supplemented anamnesis with the intermediate technique of interpretation he came to the conclusion that there were other curative factors. The concept of 'insight', however, is Adlerian. Like Adler, Rogers thinks that the patient benefits from a clear recognition of all her motives, feelings and attitudes, and from a clear understanding of the reasons why she is behaving as she does and why she has her particular symptoms. This process of recognizing and understanding is not of course purely intellectual, as he points out;

it is bound to disturb the patient emotionally. But the process is primarily intellectual, and both Adler and Rogers regard it as the most important of the curative factors. The third factor—the natural potentiality for recovery—is one which he has only recently recognized.[1] If the counsellor is able to refrain from 'direction', and concentrate on assisting the client to achieve catharsis and insight, this will release the 'potentiality of the individual for constructive action'. This is reminiscent of the belief in the '*vis medicatrix naturae*' which seems to me to be an underlying assumption of the Freudians' technique, but is not so clearly stated by them.

Rogers' technique consists, essentially, of inducing the patient to talk as freely as possible about all aspects of her symptoms or difficulties. This is achieved by a conversation in which the counsellor tries to induce the patient to do most of the talking, while he confines himself to remarks which will either encourage her to express herself more freely or help her to appreciate the significance of what she has been saying. He thus uses a gentle form of interpretation, which does not suggest to the patient that she has unconscious motives quite different from her conscious ones, but merely repeats what she has been saying in words that make her see more clearly the implications of what she has been saying. Rogers' form of interpretation is thus much less authoritative and suggestive than that of the Adlerian or neo-Freudian psychotherapist, who will often use 'forced interpretation' to compel the patient to recognize and face feelings and motives that she is not yet ready to express herself.

The topics which form the subject of the patient's conversation with the psychotherapist are therefore her choice rather than his, whereas the Freudian or Adlerian psychotherapist tends to steer the conversation in certain directions which he considers beneficial. As a result, the topics chosen by Rogers' patients are much more varied and more closely connected with the symptoms which brought them to him than the topics to which Freudians or Adlerians devote so much time.

Like Adler, Rogers makes no effort to induce anamnesis of the patient's childhood experiences; nor does he make any use of dream-interpretation, or free association. As for transference, he recognizes the occurrence of the phenomenon, but he does not attempt to use it to further his therapeutic ends. He regards the

[1] In *Client-centered Therapy*, 1951.

patient's 'positive' or 'negative' feelings as really directed towards the process of treatment, which may be pleasant or unpleasant at that particular stage, and not towards the counsellor himself. Rogers also recognizes (and uses the term) 'resistance'—that is the patient's involuntary unco-operativeness in treatment; but unlike the Freudians he does not believe that it is an inevitable phenomenon of treatment, and attributes it to unskilful handling of the patient by the counsellor; he thinks, for example, that it is usually due to a premature attempt by the counsellor to force an unwelcome interpretation down a patient's throat.

Like orthodox psychoanalysts Rogers now considers that the counsellor should avoid giving the patient advice on the conduct of her life outside the consulting-room. Indeed, just as Freud's technique was very largely shaped by the fear of inadvertently employing any form of the suggestive method out of which it grew, so Rogers' is at pains to emphasize the difference between what he calls 'non-directive therapy' and the 'directive' method from which it is descended, with its positive advice about everyday conduct. He also resembles orthodox Freudians in believing that friendship or even social contact between counsellor and client is undesirable.

Unlike most psychoanalysts, on the other hand, Rogers does not consider that 'interviews', as he calls them, should be very frequent. He thinks that they should be several days, or a week, apart, in order that the 'client' should assimilate what has been achieved in the last interview. In this he resembles Jung. His results appear to be achieved in a very much shorter time than is claimed by most psychoanalysts; he actually estimates that only 'six to fifteen contacts' are normally necessary. Unlike Freudians and Jungians, he does not insist on a personal analysis as an essential in the training of a counsellor; he believes that provided that the counsellor is a person who combines a reasonable sensitivity to human feelings with a certain amount of objectivity and self-understanding, it is sufficient for him to acquire the necessary skill through lectures in psychological and sociological subjects and through supervised experience of actual counselling.

Rogers' non-directive counselling is thus interesting for two reasons. Historically, it appears to simplify the Freudian technique even further than Adler's did, although it avoids his argumentative method of forcing interpretation on his patients, and lacks most

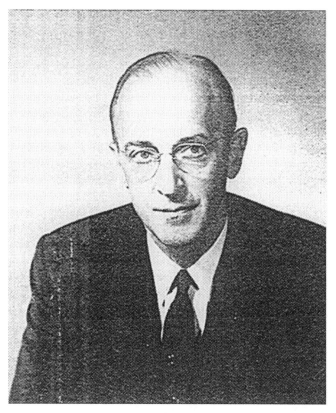

Carl Roger.

of the concepts of the Freudian or Adlerian explanatory models. Indeed, its very lack of such concepts is the other point of interest. As a result of its highly empirical origins it seems to have developed without the heavy superstructure of technical terms and explanatory models that are such a marked feature of psychoanalysis. At the same time, the importance which it attaches to catharsis reflects the early Freudian point of view, although it shares the Adlerian emphasis on insight and the Adlerian neglect of the anamnesis of childhood experiences.

Recommended Reading

ALFRED ADLER, by Hertha Orgler. C. W. Daniels.

ALFRED ADLER, by Lewis Way. Pelican Books, 1956.

INDIVIDUAL PSYCHOLOGY, by Alfred Adler. Kegan Paul, 1925.

COUNSELLING AND PSYCHOTHERAPY, by Carl Rogers. Houghton Mifflin, 1942.

THE DEVELOPMENT OF CLIENT-CENTERED THERAPY IN THE WRITINGS OF CARL ROGERS, by Dell Lebo, in the *American Journal of Psychiatry*, 1953.

V

ANALYTICAL PSYCHOLOGY— DEVELOPMENT AND THEORY

JUNG'S ASSOCIATION WITH FREUD

CARL GUSTAV JUNG (1875–) is the son of a Swiss pastor and philologist. He was educated and took his medical degree at Basle, and in 1900 became an assistant to Bleuler at the Burghölzli Mental Hospital at Zürich, where he was a colleague of Karl Abraham (see Chapter VII). Soon after he also became an assistant at the psychiatric clinic of Zürich University, and in 1905 he was appointed lecturer in psychology to the University itself.

The publication of Freud's *Interpretation of Dreams* in 1900 attracted the attention of Bleuler and Jung. Bleuler had taken part in hypnotic experiments under the influence of the French school, and as early as 1898 Jung had been interested in the psychology of so-called 'occult' phenomena. After the publication of Freud's book he seems to have decided to follow Freud's example and visit Paris, which he did in 1902. In that year he published a thesis on 'The Psychology and Pathology of Occult Phenomena', in which the influence of the Parisian school of psychologists, and particularly Janet, is very marked. Their studies of curiosities such as automatic writing, hysterical somnambulism and multiple personality had led them to the conception of unconscious personalities which could at times take over the control of the body from the conscious personality. Jung used this explanation to account for as many of his phenomena as he could, but concludes by saying that there are some which are very hard to explain in this way; we shall see later how this affected his attitude towards psychoanalysis. On his return to the Burghölzli, however, he began to study the concept of the unconscious from another point of view. One of the subjects which Galton and the Leipzig psychologists (chiefly Wundt and Cattell) had been studying for a quarter of a century was 'word-associations'. If you draw up a list of words—such as 'head; green; water; sing' and so on, and say them one by one to someone, asking him to reply with the first word that comes into his mind, the results will vary surprisingly with different people. In the first place, the words suggested to them by the stimulus-words will be very different. Secondly, some words will, for no obvious reason, make this person or that pause a long time before they can think of a response-word; some people will even fail completely to produce one. Jung's study suggested that these dissimilarities, and particularly the time-intervals, were indications not so much of intellectual variations (although of course certain types of response were typical of mental deficiency or other cerebral impairment) as of differences in the individual's emotional reaction towards subjects connected with the stimulus-word. For example, a nurse in his hospital who had stolen money took much longer than her innocent colleagues to react to words connected with the theft. Moreover, he observed abnormal reactions in neurotics which had no discernible connection with their conscious emotional attitudes but which were closely connected with emotions or experiences which they revealed only after searching questions or even treatment of the psychoanalytic type. This was regarded as a striking experimental confirmation of Freud's clinical conception of repressed and unconscious mental phenomena.

Bleuler and Jung were now in correspondence with Freud, and in 1906 the three met at the Salzburg conference of the Psychoanalytical Association. Freud and Jung took a strong liking to each other, and as a result of this meeting Jung was made editor, under the joint direction of Freud and Bleuler, of the Association's journal. In 1909 Freud, Jung and Ferenczi paid a joint visit to the United States in order to lecture at Worcester College, Massachusetts; it was during this visit that Jung hinted to the young Ernest Jones that he found the Freudian practice of discussing sex and other unsavoury topics with patients both embarrassing and unnecessary. He later allowed Freud, however, to make him President of the Association, and it was not until 1912, a year after the break with Adler, that Freud realized the danger of a second secession. Bleuler had already withdrawn from the Association, ostensibly because it was against his principles to belong to an international body, and was writing alternate defences and criticisms of psychoanalysis: both Freud and Jung were finding it difficult to keep on good terms with him. As Ernest Jones points out, however, it is very difficult for a Swiss to run counter to public opinion in his small and closely knit country, and psychoanalysis, after the intense interest which always greeted it at first, had given great offence, through its preoccupation with sexual matters, to the strict and Calvinistic Protestantism which prevails there. Jung, as we have seen, had been uneasy about this aspect for several years, and in 1913 he resigned the editorship of the journal, saying that no further co-operation with Freud was possible.[1] Early in 1914 he resigned the Presidency of the Association. His own theories and technique have since been distinguished from Freud's by the name of 'Analytical Psychology'.

JUNG'S DIFFERENCES FROM FREUD

The extent to which the two strong personalities contributed to this schism is still being debated; but our concern is with the theoretical and even more the technical differences between them. We have seen that, like Adler, Jung objected to the embarrassment of discussing sexual matters with his patients. At the same time he was convinced of the efficacy of the Freudian technique in dealing with certain types of patient (although, as we shall see, there were other types for which he considered it unsuitable). Yet this technique seemed to involve a concentration on sexual matters. This might to some extent be due, he thought, to the bias of the psychoanalyst himself; but this could not be the whole truth, for his own patients had a tendency to dwell on such topics. Part of the explanation, he thought, was the therapeutic effect of confessing any burdensome secret, of whatever nature; in the case of many patients this happened to be sexual. It is interesting to notice here how close he was to Fromm's theory that the Freudian insistence on sex and aggression as fundamental springs of action arose from the effect of a particular kind of social organization upon its members, and might not be true of other cultures (see Chapter VII). But Jung's solution was more like that of Adler, who explained the

[1] In the same year he gave up his psychiatric teaching at the University of Zürich, but the connection between this and his secession from Freud is not clear to me.

importance of sexual motivation by saying that it was simply one manifestation of the patient's striving for power and domination. Jung regarded it as a manifestation of a general psychic energy, to which he gave the name of libido. Freud had, of course, used this term before he met Jung, but in the sense in which it was used by nineteenth-century medical schools, that is, as meaning sexual desire. Under Jung's influence he came to use it in a rather wider sense, so that it meant the psychic energy which provided the motive power for all pleasure-seeking behaviour; but it is doubtful whether he ever regarded it as the power-source for the aggressive instinct. For Jung, on the other hand, it was the source of all behaviour, aggressive or pleasure-seeking. As he himself appreciated, it was a psychological version of Bergson's biological conception of the *élan vital*. While there are thus differences between the form which the concept of libido took in the explanatory models of Jung and Freud, they are highly theoretical differences. Their practical effect on technique was that in treating an abnormality that had no obviously sexual features Freud would not be satisfied until he had induced the patient to recall and talk freely about his infantile sexual development; while Jung, though not excluding discussion of sexual matters, would not insist that they must be involved. Moreover, if the discussion did turn upon them he would not accept them as the ultimate explanation but would try to see why the libido had taken that particular turn. It is no condemnation of his technique to point out that this feature of it has unfortunately proved attractive to some neurotics for the wrong reason, namely that they hope to avoid dwelling on their sexual difficulties.

The second factor that contributed to the differences in Jung's theory was his interest in mythology. He had shared the interest of Janet and other French psychologists in the phenomena of dissociation. Certain people are prone to states in which they say or write words, or perform other actions, without afterwards being able to recall or explain them. Examples of dissociation are automatic writing, multiple personality and the trances of 'mediums'. It was in the last of these groups that Jung took most interest, and most of his thesis on 'The Psychology and Pathology of Occult Phenomena' consists of a detailed account of séances with the fifteen-year-old daughter of a Protestant clergyman. While he succeeded in tracing most of what she said to books that she was known to have read, he was struck by the similarity between its general pattern and that of several occultist works that were quite inaccessible to her. Later, when he was in charge of psychotic patients at the Burghölzli, he noticed how many of their delusions or hallucinations not only repeated the same theme (there was, for example, the well-known tendency to believe that one is God, or the mother of all mankind) but also recalled old myths. Most striking of all was the patient who, in her quieter moments, described some really unusual visions and images to Jung in 1906. In 1910 Jung came across a Greek papyrus dealing with similar material which had only recently been deciphered and thus could not have been known to his patient. These observations led him, between 1913 and 1917, to modify the Freudian notion of the unconscious in an important way. Like Freud, he seems to have found the years of the first world war a time for the revision of his theoretical concepts, and he embarked on an even more intensive study of mythology and primitive ways of thinking. This not only involved him in the reading of an astonishing range of works, from the writings of the mediaeval alchemists and more modern mystics to the translations of Chinese and other oriental philosophers; but also took him, after the war, on personal expeditions to primitive societies in New Mexico, North Africa, Kenya, India, England and the United States.

Both Freud and Jung came to use the concept of the unconscious as a result of their contact with the French investigators of hysteria and dissociation. But Freud, before he was influenced by Jung, regarded the contents of the unconscious as consisting entirely of the memories, phantasies, desires and emotions that the individual had repressed in the course of her childhood. Jung came to believe that the unconscious also contained things that could not be traced to any experience of that individual but could be traced to the experience of earlier generations of human beings. He pointed, for example, to the way in which not only psychotic delusions and hallucinations but also the dreams of non-psychotics resembled myths which were hundreds of years old and which in some cases were not known to the individual; and he also drew attention—as of course others had before him—to the close resemblance between the myths of societies in widely separated parts of the world. Freud believed, of course, that the structure of the mind, with its divisions into the conscious, perceiving, reasoning part and the unconscious, irrational part, had come about as the consequence of a long process of evolution; and under Jung's influence he admitted that certain primitive ways of thinking and feeling—such as the son's hostility to his father and attachment to his mother—might be a survival in modern man of a reaction that was more appropriate to a very primitive stage of social organization, when men lived in separate families, with one male possessing all the women (see Chapter VII). He also believed that the similarities between the working of individual minds could be used to explain the odd and irrational behaviour of crowds and other large groups of men under the domination of a leader. His anthropological studies—such as *Totem and Taboo* (1913)—recognized the similarity between certain primitive ways of thinking and the neurotic's defence-mechanisms.

There are, however, only two ways in which Freud's therapeutic technique makes use of the assumption of psychological inheritance, and even these were probably not clearly recognized by him in this light. In the first place, his intermediate technique of interpretation, which makes use of such notions as repression, rationalization, displacement, sublimation and the other 'defence-mechanisms', implies that the minds of all patients work in very much the same way. Some of course may be more prone than others to rationalization, others to sublimation; but all the defence-mechanisms, he assumes, can be seen at work in every mind. In addition to this inherited similarity in the way in which the human mind deals with its difficulties, his method of interpretation also implies an inherited connection between the contents of some of our thoughts. For his notion of 'symbolism' allowed him to interpret images from dreams and phantasies on the assumption that a given image always represents the same thing in the unconscious minds of different people. Thus a dream-snake always stands for a penis, whether the dreamer be man or woman, and whether he has ever seen a real snake in his life. This assumption that there is a universal symbolic glossary implies that our minds have inherited not only the trick of symbolizing but also the symbols themselves.

THE PERSONAL UNCONSCIOUS

These technical assumptions were scarcely recognized by Freud, but were very strongly emphasized by Jung. He divided the unconscious into two parts, the 'personal' and the 'collective'. The personal unconscious is formed from

(i) the desires, emotions and impulses that the individual has repressed in his childhood;

(ii) 'lost memories', which include, in addition to those inaccessible through repression, memories of experiences that left too faint an impression to be recalled under normal circumstances;

(iii) 'subliminal perceptions'—that is, sense-impressions that are too faint to become conscious: this is not a very important item from Jung's point of view, and while he probably means sense-impressions that are taking place at the moment, and not past ones (which would belong to item (ii)), he does not say so clearly;

(iv) 'contents that are not yet ripe for consciousness', by which he means certain potentialities of the individual's character which he is unable to realize.

The important items in this list are the first and the last. It will be seen that in (i) Jung has adopted Freud's explanatory model of repressed mental phenomena, but in (iv) has added something of a rather different nature. His experience of psychotics at the Burghölzli had suggested that in spite of the variety of their symptoms there was one fundamental difference between them and hysterics, and in 1913 he tried to define this.

It is well known that in their general physiognomy hysteria and dementia praecox present a striking contrast, which is seen particularly in the attitude of the sufferers towards the external world. The reactions provoked in the hysteric surpass the normal level of intensity of feeling, whilst this level is not reached at all by the precocious dement. The picture presented by these contrasted illnesses is one of exaggerated emotivity in the one, and extreme apathy in the other, with regard to the environment. In their personal relations this is very marked. . . . All this clearly indicates that hysteria is characterized by a centrifugal tendency of the libido, whilst in dementia praecox its tendency is centripetal. . . . I propose to use the terms 'extroversion' and 'introversion' to describe these two opposite directions of the libido. . . .[1]

[1] 'A Contribution to the Study of Psychological Types', delivered at the Munich Psychoanalytical Congress, 1913 (tr. C. E. Long). Most Jungians spell 'extraversion' correctly.

Although this distinction was based on his observation of pathological individuals, Jung came to the conclusion that even normal people could be classified either as extraverts or as introverts. The former are sociable, quick to react to situations, and tend to welcome and adjust themselves more readily to new developments. The introvert, on the other hand, enjoys being alone, or with a single friend; his automatic reaction to a new development is withdrawal; his judgment is more independent of public opinion, and he 'lives with his thoughts'. Jung found a rough recognition of his two 'attitude-types' in the writings of such men as William James; he had classified philosophers into the 'tender-minded', who are interested only in 'the inner life and spiritual things', and the 'tough-minded', who lay most stress on 'material things and objective reality'. This part of Jung's theory is more easily testable than most of the rest, and it is interesting to find that the tough-minded statistician-psychologist H. J. Eysenck, who is extremely sceptical of most psychotherapeutic concepts, has satisfied himself by tests that there is a factor, quite separate from those of neuroticism and psychoticism, which seems to make it necessary to place every individual somewhere on an 'introversion-extraversion' scale.[1]

During the first world war, however, Jung elaborated this distinction considerably by sub-dividing both extraverts and introverts into four 'function-types'. The notion of a four-fold classification of human beings was even older than the notion of a two-fold one, for Galen's medicine had based a type-classification on its explanatory model of 'humours'; a man was 'choleric', 'sanguine', 'phlegmatic' or 'melancholic', according to the humour which was supposed to be most plentiful in his body. Jung's innovation consisted in his choice of four 'functions' on which to base his classification. They are

(i) *sensation:* most of the 'sensation type's' behaviour is governed by the senses. Jung does not include only 'sensualists' in this category; he is also referring to people who take the evidence of their senses at its face value, without doubting it or exercising any reason or imagination upon it; who regard a spade as a spade.

(ii) *intuition:* like sensation types, intuitive people are also irrational, but unlike them they can look beyond the mere facts

[1] *Dimensions of Personality*, 1947.

of a situation, and can diagnose its causes and envisage what can be made of it. Scientists, physicians, inventors, and some politicians belong to this group.

(iii) *feeling:* by this Jung means the function of attaching values to things and situations. This gives rise of course to emotional reactions towards them, but the feeling function is distinct from these emotions. People with very definite ideas as to what is right and wrong, what is good or bad art, which acquaintances are friends and enemies, belong to this type. Their ideas on these subjects are systematic, reasoned and hard to alter.

(iv) *thinking:* the thinker deals in ideas; he not only reasons logically but also has imagination; he likes to find formulae in which to systematize the facts or express his speculations. It is the thinking type who is responsible for new ways of thought; examples are Newton, Einstein, Descartes.

Jung visualizes these functions as the four points of the compass, with sensation at the opposite pole to intuition, and feeling opposed to thinking. On top of this fourfold classification he super-imposes a broad division of human beings into the two 'attitude-types' —the 'introverted' and the 'extraverted'. Thus any of Jung's four function-types can be either introverted or extraverted, so that his two classifications yield eight types—introverted thinkers, extraverted thinkers, introverted intuitives and so on. Frieda Fordham has given some excellent sketches of all eight types in men and women.[1] There is undoubtedly a great deal of acute observation in this classification. It is, however, one of the parts of Jung's theory that ought to be capable of verification by experimental psychologists, and they have had difficulty in finding support for the theory of function-types.

However that may be, Jung not only believed that everyone belonged to one of these eight types, but made this classification the basis of what is, logically, an even more interesting theory. He decided that an introvert must also have an extraverted side of which he was not conscious and to which he was not giving any scope, and *vice versa.* What was more, a thinker was giving too little expression to his other three functions, namely feeling, sensa-

[1] In *An Introduction to Jung's Psychology,* 1953; a more diffuse account will be found in Jung's own *Psychological Types* (1920).

tion and intuition; while each of the other function-types was also failing to give free play to the other three functions. Together with the individual's repressed desires these were the important contents of the personal unconscious, the 'contents not yet ripe for consciousness', and one of the objects of his therapeutic technique must be to induce the patient to give them equal scope with all the other functions.

This is a very good example of a theory which by the standards of the scientist or logician is paradoxical and almost self-contradictory. Assuming for the sake of argument that the classification itself is based upon sound observation, the logician might say that its whole point is that people belong to one or other of these classes, and to talk of the other functions as being 'unconscious' is to say that in some way they really belong to all the classes. What Jung seems to have done is to take a classification which belongs to the observations of what I called 'natural history' in Chapter I, and then to turn it into an explanatory model of what I called the 'life-like' kind by talking as if the classes to which the patient does not belong were unconscious entities of the same nature as Freud's model of repressed desires and memories.

Jung might reply, however, that he is not a scientist trying to explain or predict, but a technician trying to improve his patient's condition; and that it does improve it to develop the undeveloped functions. If it is in fact possible to develop them (and Jung thinks that it is) then it is technically convenient (even if illogical) to think of these potentialities as part of the patient, in order to distinguish them from all the functions that the patient cannot be expected to develop—such as levitation.

THE COLLECTIVE UNCONSCIOUS

The collective unconscious is Jung's name for all the ways of thinking and behaving, and all the contents of our thoughts, that human beings inherit from earlier generations. A good example is the way in which young children who have never seen a lion or tiger outside a picture-book or the cage of a zoo, and thus have no individual experience of their ferocity, will have nightmares about them. In order to have the nightmare about a tiger it is probably necessary that the child should see either the animal itself or a picture of it; but the fear with which the image of the animal is henceforth endowed seems to be contributed by the child without any personal experience to justify it. Jung, of course, goes further than this; his chief justification for the concept of the collective unconscious is the close similarity which he sees between a patient's dreams and the themes of common myths. One of the commonest of these themes is that of a hero, who is a sun-god in some form, and journeys, enclosed in a boat or box, over the sea by night, encountering various dangers. He is sometimes accompanied by a woman. At the end of the journey he escapes. Examples of this sort of myth which leap to the mind are Jonah and the Whale, Kipling's shipwrecked mariner 'of infinite resource and sagacity', Hiawatha, Osiris, Odysseus and several seafaring saints. There can of course be few patients who have not come across this sort of myth in their own reading, even if they cannot remember having done so; but Jung believes that this is not necessary, and that some patients' dreams are modelled on myths which not they but their ancestors learned.

The notion of inherited memory was not invented by Jung. As early as 1870 Professor Ewald Hering,[1] the Viennese physiologist, had suggested that memory was a function of all organic matter, and could be inherited in the same way as the colour of one's hair. At first sight this seems to imply the somewhat doubtful Lamarckian doctrine of the inheritance of acquired characteristics, in which Hering himself certainly believed; but Jung and his followers deny that their theory has this implication. It is of course possible that a particular way of thinking, like a bird's method of nest-building, are transmissible characteristics but are inherited in a Darwinian and not a Lamarckian way; this might happen because those who do not think in that way have less chance of reproducing themselves. This is quite plausible, since people who think in a noticeably different way from the rest of their community have difficulty in finding mates, and may even be outlawed completely. But if Jungians mean, as they sometimes seem to, that they do not believe in the inheritance of ways of thought by either Darwinian or Lamarckian means, they can be relying only on a rather mystical idea of the collective unconscious as subsisting by itself, independent of human beings. Certainly some Jungians seem to think that under its influence a person can think and behave in ways learned not by him or any of his ancestors but by someone who may have

[1] Whose theories were known to Freud and therefore probably to Jung.

no descendants left—for example that an Aberdonian of pure Caucasian blood may be influenced by Inca legends of which neither he nor his forebears have ever heard.

ARCHETYPES

Some images of particular importance occur frequently, not only in the dreams, phantasies and hallucinations of patients but also in literature and the arts. These Jung called 'primordial images' at first, a phrase borrowed from his history professor at Basle, Jakob Burckhardt; but he soon adopted the term 'archetypes', a word used by St. Augustine to describe Plato's eternal 'ideas'. 'The archetype', Jung says, 'is a kind of readiness to produce over and over again the same or similar mythical ideas.' Since the archetype is a way of thinking, and not a single idea, it is usually symbolized in our conscious thought by concrete images, which may take different forms but have a recognizable common element. One of the simpler archetypes is described by Jung in these words:

One of the archetypes that is almost invariably met with in the projection of unconscious collective contents is the 'magic demon' with mysterious powers. A good example of this is Gustav Meyrink's *Golem*, also the Tibetan wizard in the same author's *Fledermäuse*, who unleashes world war by magic. . . . The magician type also figures in *Zarathustra*, while in *Faust* he is the actual hero.

The image of this demon forms one of the lowest and most ancient stages in the conception of God. It is the type of primitive tribal sorcerer or medicine-man, a peculiarly gifted personality endowed with magical power. This figure often appears as dark-skinned and of mongoloid type, and then it represents a negative and possibly dangerous aspect. . . . .

The recognition of the archetypes takes us a long step forward. The magical or daemonic effect emanating from our neighbour disappears when the mysterious feeling is traced back to a definite entity in the collective unconscious.

It is of course conceivable that the 'magic demon' archetype might never occur among the dream- or phantasy-images of a particular patient. But there are other archetypes which must inevitably be encountered, since they represent universal aspects of the human psyche. These are

(i) the *persona:* every human being who lives in a society in-
    stinctively compromises between his real nature and the
    part which society expects him to play. 'A businessman
    will try to appear (and even to be) forceful and energetic, a
    professional man intelligent, a civil servant correct . . . a
    wife is required to be a hostess, a mother, a partner or
    whatever her husband's position demands.'[1] Poseurs are
    people who overdevelop their persona; those who are un-
    able to develop it sufficiently are regarded as gauche or
    'unpredictable'.

(ii) the *shadow:* this is the part of ourselves which we do not
    like, the 'underside' of our personality, as it were. The
    shadow of an upright, civilized, correct professional man
    like Dr. Jekyll will be a primitive, immoral, unscrupulous,
    murdering brute like Mr. Hyde. Since it is our way of
    thinking about all our repressed desires and attitudes, Jung
    rather loosely says that it *is* the personal unconscious, al-
    though as we have seen the personal unconscious includes
    more than the repressed. The shadow is symbolized in
    dreams, phantasies and literature by an inferior or primitive
    person or by someone whom we know and dislike.

(iii) the *imago:* like Freud, Jung thought that the unconscious
    of man contains a complementary female element, the
    anima, while that of woman contains a male element, the
    animus. This is manifested not only in the so-called
    feminine traits which even the most virile man betrays at
    times (and *vice versa*), but also in the role which he expects
    the women in his life—his mother, his wife, his daughters—
    to play. This role is partly determined by his childhood
    experience of his mother (as Freud pointed out, men's
    attitude to their wives is often to be traced to their mothers)
    but also, to a very important extent, by the experience of
    generations of men with women.

Other archetypes may manifest themselves. Men may visualize
themselves as 'the old wise man': if for one reason or another they
are able to use the inherited experience of the collective uncon-

[1] Frieda Fordham, loc. cit.

scious, they may make the mistake of crediting themselves with almost magical wisdom, including prophetic powers. Mystics, politicians, television pundits and asylum inmates who think they are God are manifestations of this archetype. Women, particularly masculine ones, can also behave in this way; but women are more likely to see themselves as 'the great mother'.

Anyone possessed by this figure comes to believe herself endowed with an infinite capacity for loving and understanding, helping and protecting, and will wear herself out in the service of others. She can however also be most destructive, insisting (though not necessarily openly) that all who come within her circle of influence are 'her children', and therefore helpless or dependent on her in some degree. This subtle tyranny, if carried to extremes, can demoralize and destroy the personality of others.[1]

It is possible to see in notions such as the *persona*, the *shadow* and the *imago* the influence of Jung's early interest in the French studies of dissociation. Not only are many of the human figures of our dreams supposed to stand for these parts of our personalities, but the parts themselves are described by Jung and his followers as if they were almost complete personalities, although of a one-sided kind. The cases studied by the Paris school included quite a few in which the subject temporarily assumed a second personality, markedly different from the normal one. Sometimes the subject could recall in her normal state the words and actions of her second personality, sometimes not. The schoolgirl who was the principal theme of Jung's thesis also exhibited mediumistic states which bordered on dissociation of this kind. In more than one case this dissociation seemed to have begun at puberty, a stage of rapid development in both body and personality, and in at least two cases quoted by Jung the secondary personality eventually replaced the normal one. He says, for example, that his schoolgirl gradually turned into the mature and capable woman who had been one of her 'spirit guides'. Jung therefore concluded that 'It is not unthinkable that the phenomena of double consciousness are nothing but the character formations for the future personality, or their attempt to burst forth'.[2]

[1] Frieda Fordham, loc. cit.
[2] *On the Psychology and Pathology of so-called Occult Phenomena*, 1902.

Unlike the contents of the personal unconscious, which can be made conscious by the removal of repression (in the case of desires and suchlike) or by being developed (in the case of 'functions'), the contents of the collective unconscious cannot be made conscious. Jung and his followers often attribute this to its ancient origins and the wide difference between its nature and that of the conscious mind. Jung says of the archetypes, 'indeed not even our thought can clearly grasp them, for it never invented them'. It is obvious, however, that the impossibility of making them conscious is not so much a practical as a logical impossibility, and Jung sometimes seems almost to recognize this. The contents of the collective unconscious are not thoughts but a tendency to have certain thoughts—as Jung himself says, 'a kind of readiness to produce over and over again the same or similar mythical ideas'; you cannot think a tendency in the same way as you can think a thought; all you can do is to think a thought that is an example of that tendency. In the same way, you can feel rain, snow and frost, but not the cold climate of which they are the instances. A clear idea of the logical status of Jung's collective unconscious would not only dispel some of the rather mystical awe with which some of his followers regard it, but would also reconcile quite a few of the sceptics, who imagine that he believes in something as real as our conscious thoughts, shared by everyone and yet accessible to no one, like the bottom of the Pacific outside territorial waters. This reification of a mere tendency is, I think, a mistake of some Jungians but not of Jung himself.

Recommended Reading

PROFESSOR C. G. JUNG, by Michael Fordham, in the *British Journal of Medical Psychology*, 1945.

AN INTRODUCTION TO JUNG'S PSYCHOLOGY, by Frieda Fordham. Pelican Books, 1953.

ANALYTICAL PSYCHOLOGY, by C. G. Jung, tr. edited by C. E. Long. Baillière, Tindall, and Cox, 1920.

VI

ANALYTICAL PSYCHOLOGY—
TECHNIQUE

BEFORE going on to consider the connection between the theory and technique of analytical psychology, it is worth noting one or two points. In the first place, Jung himself does not put forward his technique as a rival to Freud's for all types of case. He distinguishes four kinds of patient. There are those 'who just want sound common sense and good advice. With luck they can be disposed of in a single consultation.' Next there is the patient 'for whom a thorough confession or abreaction is enough'. Thirdly, 'the severer neuroses usually require a reductive analysis of their symptoms and states. And here one should not apply this or that method indiscriminately but, according to the nature of the case, should conduct the analysis more along the lines of Freud or more along those of Adler. . . . There are in fact two categories of people with different needs. . . .'[1]

These three categories generally account, in Jung's view, for the younger neurotic patient—that is, the patient under forty years of age. He finds his own technique of most value with older patients. What is more, he says

> The clinical material at my disposal is of a peculiar composition; new cases are decidedly in the minority. Most of them already have some form of psychotherapeutic treatment behind them, with partial or negative results. About a third of my cases are not suffering from any clinically definable neurosis, but from the senselessness and aimlessness of their lives. . . . Fully two-thirds of my patients are in the second half of life.

[1] 'Principles of Practical Psychotherapy', 1935 (*Collected Works*, Vol. 16).

Certainly, irrespective of the merits of Jung's own particular technique, it seems reasonable to argue that the neurotic in 'the second half of life' may call for a different technique. Even the most fanatical Freudian would admit that the older a patient is when she begins treatment the slower, more difficult and less complete is the therapeutic process. What is more, there comes a time in the lives of both men and women—although the exact age may vary very greatly—at which purely physiological changes reduce the strength and importance of sexual feelings, on which orthodox psychoanalysis still lays considerable emphasis.

It is, of course, difficult to be sure to what extent Jung's innovations in technique were evolved in order to deal with the older neurotic, and to what extent they were shaped by purely theoretical considerations and then found to be of more use with this kind of patient. Freud's technical innovations were developed empirically in the course of his clinical practice, and most—though unfortunately not all—of his theoretical concepts were evolved out of them. Jung's early clinical material, the psychotics of the Burghölzli, must have been anything but suitable subjects for experiments with psychotherapeutic methods, and most of the cases whose treatment he discusses were in fact private neurotic outpatients, whom he treated at a later date. During his formative period, therefore--that is, from about 1900 to about 1915—his ideas were probably being shaped quite as much by other influences as by his clinical successes and failures. These other influences included of course Freud; in spite of Jung's rather unscientific revulsion from the topics which Freud insisted on discussing with his patients, he based his method on Freud's, as he himself is the first to point out. But he thus took over the Freudian technique as a second-hand instrument, rather than one whose uses he had studied and understood in practice. Moreover, he relied to a great extent on sources even further divorced from direct clinical experience. His wide mythological reading, as we have seen, influenced him strongly; so did his first-hand acquaintance with primitive cultures in various parts of the world. Last, and probably least, was the influence of the world of academic psychology, to which he also belonged. We can see this in his word-association tests, and—more important—in his eight-fold classification of people into 'psychological types'; but even the latter is based on his study of earlier psychological writers—from the Gnostics to

William James—and on his everyday impressions of people, rather than on clinical or experimental observations of his own. On the whole, therefore, his technique probably owes a good deal less than Freud's to the trial and error of clinical practice. Certainly it has not been modified, either by Jung himself or his followers, to nearly the same extent as Freud modified his methods. Jungians may argue that this is because it needed less modification, particularly since Freud's early errors enabled it to start at the advanced stage where he left off; but I do not think that this completely explains the absence of further development.

Several things make it difficult to form a clear impression of the intermediate techniques which Jungians actually employ. One is the diffuseness and vagueness of the few papers which deal with such practical questions—a feature of Jung's writings which some of his followers have emulated. This is not insuperable, however, and a more serious difficulty is Jung's belief that the essence of his method is the avoidance of any set procedures. Freud, as we have seen, went to considerable lengths to avoid any taint of 'suggestion': but Jung goes even further, and says, 'Suggestion therapy includes all methods that arrogate to themselves, and apply, a knowledge of or an interpretation of other individualities. Equally it includes all strictly technical methods, because these invariably assume that all individuals are alike.'[1] Because of the uniquenesss of the individual, Jung says that the psychotherapist's only really satisfactory course is to 'confine himself to a purely dialectical procedure, adopting the attitude that shuns all methods'. In fact, however, we find him using intermediate techniques and facilitants derived from Freud and Adler, and his 'dialectical procedure' has only two really distinctive features. It is more flexible than those of Freud or Adler; the Jungian is more ready to vary his methods to suit the particular patient. But his procedure also lays more emphasis on the interaction between patient and psychotherapist and on the beneficial effects of the psychotherapist's own personality: the best example of this is in the Jungian attitude towards transference. Both these features seem to me excellent in principle (although they can obviously be overdone), and are to be found—perhaps as a result of Jung's unacknowledged influence—among the neo-Freudians (see Chapter VII); but they do not amount to new intermediate techniques.

[1] Loc. cit.

Jung's theory was that his patients were suffering from one or more of the following troubles:

(i) a need for confession of their repressed desires and memories; this could of course be dealt with by the cathartic method, and was seldom, if ever, the whole story in the case of his older neurotics;

(ii) a failure to accept and fit into their lives the ways of thinking and behaving that Jung attributed to the archetypes; Dr. Jekyll, for example, was suffering from Mr. Hyde;

(iii) the neglect of the undeveloped functions and aspects of their personalities: an introvert was suffering from lack of extraversion, and a thinker was suffering from failure to develop sensation, feeling and intuition.

To remedy these defects he employed the following intermediate techniques.

RE-EDUCATION

We have already seen, in Chapter IV, how Jung as well as Adler condemned the Freudian explanation of symptoms as 'causal', and emphasized the need for a 'purposive' approach. In this Jung went a stage further than Adler, who had merely tended to regard neurotic symptoms as means of escape from an intolerable situation or of dominating people in an indirect way. Jung tends to look in his patient's symptoms for signs, however faint, of an effort to solve her own difficulties. Clifford Allen has illustrated the point excellently by an analogy from physical medicine. It is possible to explain the high temperature of typhoid entirely in terms of the physiological changes which follow the introduction of the typhoid bacillus into the body (this corresponds to the 'causal' explanation of the Freudians). It is also, however, possible to regard it as the body's attempt to kill the bacillus (a point of view which corresponds to Jung's approach to neurotic symptoms).[1] This approach of Jung's is particularly evident in his interpretation of his patients' dreams which occur in the course of treatment. I have not been able to find any very clear example of its application to symptoms of other kinds, and, as I have suggested in Chapter V, Jung's

[1] *Modern Discoveries in Medical Psychology*, 1938.

'purposive' viewpoint is probably a question of technical handling of the patient. In Jung's hands Adler's open effort to 're-educate' the patient becomes a more subtle procedure, although it still deserves to be regarded as an independent intermediate technique. The aim of Adler's re-education was always to steer the patient in the direction of a more 'social' way of life. Jung's theories, however, do not allow him to regard this as a solution for all types of patient. After all, some extraverts may be suffering from being too dependent on social relationships, and may require to have their introverted side developed. Thus the aim of the Jungian re-education will vary with each patient, and the Jungian psychotherapist cannot, like the Adlerian, decide *a priori* upon its direction, but must look to the patient for clues.

ANAMNESIS

Because of his attitude to the 'causal' approach of Freud, Jung is much less insistent on a thorough anamnesis of the patient's childhood, although he may of course make use of it where the patient seems to him to suffer from troubles of the kind which Freud's method was evolved to deal with. In attaching less value to anamnesis he thus resembles the cultural school of psychoanalysts in the United States (see Chapter VII). Indeed, since he believes that a child's attitude to its parents is only partly determined by what the parents themselves were like, and owes a great deal to the parent-child relationship in that particular culture through previous generations, it follows that he cannot hope to trace factors in the individual's own infancy to explain all her symptoms.

INTERPRETATION

To the orthodox Freudian, the intermediate technique of interpretation—that is, of explaining to the patient what unconscious factors are at work in her—is a regrettable necessity. Ideally, free association and anamnesis coupled with the transference would enable the patient to become conscious of these factors without this assistance. Accordingly, interpretation is used only because the patient is apparently unable to do this for herself, and even so only when she appears to have reached a stage when the interpretation will not shock her too much.[1] Jung, on the other hand, believes that it is quite impossible for the patient, without a wide knowledge of mythology and primitive ways of thinking, to understand her own thoughts, feelings and behaviour: interpretation is therefore both a practical and a theoretical necessity, and is his main intermediate technique.

DREAM-INTERPRETATION

This is particularly marked in the case of dream-interpretation, which Jung regards as a most important technical instrument. He claims that, whereas Freud treats a dream as a symbolic representation of repressed desires, it is really an attempt to compensate for the way in which the patient's conscious life fails to give full expression to all unconscious factors. This would simply be a statement of the Freudian theory in less precise terms, if it were not for Jung's belief that the personal and collective unconscious includes more than what is repressed; it also includes undeveloped functions and the unintelligible archetypes. Unlike Freud, too, he thinks that a dream is often an indication, in allegorical fashion, of what is wrong with the patient, and sometimes a warning of what the patient is likely to do: in other words, an allegorical diagnosis or prognosis. Not only is this an example of Jung's teleological approach, but it also attributes to the unconscious mind a creative intelligence which Freud would have denied that it possessed. Jung therefore thinks that it is impossible for the patient to understand, without assistance, the full meaning of her dreams, whether by free association or other means; and that the therapist must explain it to the patient, taking particular care to point out both its myth-like and its diagnostic or prognostic aspects.

FREE ASSOCIATION

Jung used his word-association test as a quick means of getting a rough idea of what the patient was repressing. He found that if he made a list of all the words to which the patient's response was either particularly slow or abnormal in some other way, it was possible to see a connection between them. Thus a patient who re-

---

[1] As we shall see, the Kleinian technique is an exception to this rule. Adler also interpreted without waiting for the patient.

sponded abnormally to such words as 'sister', 'father', 'rival', 'kill', was very probably suffering from a repressed jealousy of her sister's place in her father's affections. The ideas which were linked together in the unconscious in this way he called a 'complex', a word which Freud adopted and used in his famous notion of the 'Oedipus complex'. In his early clinical experiments Jung seems to have used the word-association test as a quick diagnostic method at the start of treatment. But he makes less use than Freud of free association proper—that is, as a means of inducing the patient to arrive herself, by an uncensored train of thought, at some idea of her repressed thoughts.

TRANSFERENCE

We have seen how Freud regarded the transference, first as an unavoidable nuisance and then as something which he could use to induce the patient to co-operate in his intermediate techniques; and how his followers have come to pay more and more attention to 'analysis' of the transference as an essential topic for interpretation. Jung attaches as much importance as any neo-Freudian to this intermediate technique. But the orthodox Freudian is at pains to make his own part in the relationship as impersonal as possible, believing that if he reacts in any way to the patient's attachment or dislike he will obscure its real nature both from the patient and himself; his aim is to see, and eventually to let the patient herself see, what imaginary role and what imaginary attitudes the patient will spontaneously ascribe to him. Jung, on the other hand, believes that the therapist can best help the patient by reacting naturally to her attitude: the technical term for the therapist's feelings towards the patient is 'counter-transference'. This does not of course mean that he should return, by word or action, her exaggerated affection or her exaggerated dislike; but he should not remain impersonal, since his own reactions will help the patient to understand hers. But to steer this very difficult course it is necessary that the therapist should thoroughly understand himself, and for this he must undergo a complete analysis. (Jung claims that it was he who suggested to Freud that every therapist should first have what has come to be called a 'training analysis'.)

PICTURE-MAKING

In addition to his considerable modifications of Freud's intermediate techniques, Jung devised one of his own, which has been adopted by some Freudians and Adlerians as well as his own followers. He induces his patients to draw, or better still to paint, the subjects of their dreams or phantasies. This is not intended to be 'occupational therapy'; it is not merely 'giving the patient something to do'. Still less are the results meant to be aesthetically satisfying, although they occasionally achieve this. The point, Jung says, is that the patient

> puts down on paper what he has passively seen, thereby turning it into a deliberate act. He is not only talking about it, he is actually doing something about it. . . . Moreover, the concrete shaping of the image enforces a continuous study of it in all its parts, so that it can develop its effects to the full. This invests the bare fantasy with an element of reality, which lends it greater weight and greater driving power.

He also claims that this practice makes the patient less dependent on the therapist, since she can paint her dreams and fantasies without consulting him. Here again it is possible, I think, to see the effect of Jung's familiarity with psychotics during his early years at the Burghölzli. Many of these patients were schizophrenics, who experience hallucinations or visual distortions of reality. If their condition is not too severe, however, they are often skilful at depicting their hallucinations on paper, and some have even achieved fame: Goya and Blake are obvious examples.[1]

INDIVIDUATION

Jung admits that in many cases he must be content with removing a great deal of the patient's repression and reconciling her to the less savoury aspects of her own personality. He believes, however, that patients of high intelligence or other outstanding ability can be helped by his method to undergo a process which he calls 'individuation'. This might be crudely defined as the full development of all their unconscious potentialities. He thinks that Freud

[1] *Psychotic Art*, by Francis Reitman, 1950, illustrates this, but shows how the work of schizophrenics usually lacks the sense of colour and structure which characterizes the work of the sane artist.

was wrong in regarding the unconscious as simply a prison in which we lock up all our undesirable and criminal propensities, and that there are also desirable ones locked up along with them. They can be set free, however, only if we are prepared to face the bad with the good. Jung's own example of this process of individuation in one of his patients (to be found in *The Integration of the Personality* (1939)) is long and obscure, and it is indeed in this part of his theories that he and his followers lay themselves most open to the suspicion of mysticism. At the risk of oversimplifying his doctrine, I suggest that his point is this. Even psychotherapy on Jungian lines, which is the only kind that can enable the patient to actualize all her potentialities, cannot dictate to her the form which this actualization will take. Psychotherapy can be a midwife to the new personality which emerges, and can make sure that it emerges as complete and undamaged as possible; but it rests with the patient to recognize what her new personality is like and to remould her life so as to suit it. If she fails to do so, she is merely a cured neurotic: if she succeeds, she has achieved 'individuation'. There is more than an echo, in this doctrine, of the notion of 'rebirth' which is found in so many religions, but it can be regarded as a valuable corrective for one danger of Freudianism. This is the underlying assumption that any unusual and eccentric feature of personality is capable not only of being explained by the past history of the patient but also, in theory at least, of being cured. Jung is, I think, pointing out that you cannot cure all the eccentricities of the individual without losing something valuable, and that the psychotherapist should be able to detect what is valuable among the patient's abnormalities, and help her to develop instead of destroying it.

MINOR POINTS OF TECHNIQUE

On minor points of technique there is less divergence than might be supposed between Jungians and Freudians. For example, we have seen that Freud at first allowed himself ordinary social relations with his patients, but soon came to the conclusion that this interfered with treatment; he wanted to retain the impersonal role which he thought proper to the consulting-room so that any thoughts or attitudes which they attributed to him could be recognized as the contributions of their own pathological imaginations.

Most modern Jungians, particularly in Britain, would agree with him, although Jung's own practice is less strict. At the same time Freud's impersonal practice of making the patient lie on a couch where she could not see him is not enforced, though it is permitted, by Jungians, who allow her to sit in a chair facing them or to walk about the room if that helps her to talk more freely. We shall see that some neo-Freudians now allow their patients the same freedom.

Jung thinks that the Freudian insistence on seeing patients four or five times a week is necessary only when treatment on Freudian lines is called for. If it is not, he is satisfied with two sessions a week, and eventually even less; he says that the patient takes more than twenty-four hours to assimilate the effects of a session, and recovers no more quickly if she is treated every day; and he points out that many patients cannot afford the full Freudian frequency. Here again we shall see that many neo-Freudians see their patients only twice a week.

Like Freud, Jung believes that the personal qualities of a psychotherapist are worth more than a medical degree, and suitable laymen are accepted as members of the various societies of Analytical Psychologists in Europe and the U.S.A.; most of them practice under medical supervision. The most important part of the training of both lay and medically qualified analytical psychologists is of course a thorough personal analysis.

Almost all Jungians are opposed to the use of hypnosis or drugs, even as facilitants for their own intermediate techniques. There are exceptions, of course. In 1953 Drs. R. A. Sandison, A. M. Spencer and J. D. A. Whitelaw reported[1] the use of lysergic acid diethylamide ('LSD') on a small sample of neurotic patients at Powick Mental Hospital in Worcestershire, England. Hitherto experiments with normal subjects had suggested that the effects of the drug were to produce a temporary psychosis, with hallucinations. In a few cases of neurosis, however, it had been observed that the drug sometimes caused the patient to relive childhood experiences, and this was confirmed by Sandison, Spencer and Whitelaw's experiment. Dr. Sandison observed that not only the revived memories but also the hallucinations bore 'a striking similarity to the dream and phantasy material of patients undergoing deep analysis (sc. on Jungian lines)'. He treated some of the patients by Jungian analysis

[1] In the *Journal of Mental Science*, 1954.

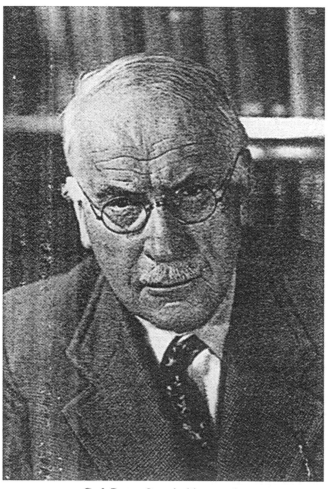

Carl Gustav Jung in his seventies.

[*to face page* 96

both during and after their periods under the influence of LSD, and found that they 'can actively influence the images produced under LSD so that they can consciously explore their minds and learn something from the great wisdom of the unconscious'.[1]

THE FUNDAMENTAL ASSUMPTIONS OF ANALYTICAL PSYCHOLOGY

I drew attention at the end of Chapter III to a number of fundamental assumptions which seemed to me to be implied in the psychoanalytic sub-technique. In the first place, psychoanalysis is *deterministic*. Jung makes a great deal of the difference between his teleological approach and Freud's causal one, but I have already argued that this boils down to the extent to which Jungians like to talk to their patients about what is going to happen, while the Freudians talk about the patients' past. I do not find in Jung anything corresponding to the metaphysical doctrine of free-will.

Nor do I find his theory any less or any more *materialistic* than Freudianism. It has, of course, been a happy play-ground for those who have sought escape from Freud's biological, deterministic, atheistic[2] approach, with its studied exploration of the most unsavoury aspects of personality and its equally studied avoidance of moral judgments. As we have seen, Jung himself was seeking an escape from the Freudian emphasis on sexuality when he seceded from Freud. But he never denied the value of the Freudian method —his one criticism is that it may not deal with the whole trouble. Some of his remarks about religious belief have been regarded as assertions of its truth; but they do not seem to me to be more than assertions of its value as an adjuvant to therapy, which neither supports nor disproves its truth.

I mentioned, however, what I called the 'egalitarianism' of the Freudian approach, which regards the new-born child as equipped simply with a set of instincts and a mental mechanism with a few parts and a tendency to certain tricks of self-defence against these instincts, such as repression. Fromm's cultural theories, which question whether the instincts as Freud described them are really innate, is even more egalitarian. For the Freudian all neurosis is

---

[1] Loc. cit.

[2] Although Freud himself was an atheist, his approach is not necessarily incompatible with Christianity.

to some extent attributable to what happens to the child after it is born. For the Jungian, on the other hand, the child is not only born with a certain constitutional disposition towards introversion or extraversion, and reliance on one of the four functions, but is also burdened from the start with ways of thinking, feeling and behaving which she inherits from her remote forebears. This would mean that Jungianism was at bottom more pessimistic than Freudianism, if it were not for Jung's belief that the patient can be enabled by treatment to fit these inherited ways of thought and feeling into her conscious life and to develop the undeveloped functions of her personality.

Recommended Reading

(in addition to books recommended in Chapter VI)

THE PRACTICE OF PSYCHOTHERAPY, by C. G. Jung. Routledge and Kegan Paul, Vol. 16 in the *Collected Works*, 1955.

VII

POST-FREUDIAN PSYCHOANALYSIS

AT the end of Chapter III I described the form which psychoanalysis assumed in the hands of Freud's close followers in the nineteen-thirties. This form still survives, and can properly be called 'orthodox psychoanalysis'. Meanwhile, however, different groups of psychoanalysts have developed variants of the Freudian technique. In doing so they have been influenced in some cases by one of the two great apostates, Adler or Jung, and in other cases by the circumstances in which they were practising. Their variants are not, however, so unlike psychoanalysis that they need be regarded as new species like those of Adler or Jung, and most of the practitioners belong to their national Psychoanalytic Association. Collectively they are known as neo-Freudians, and they fall broadly into three groups—the object-relations school, the cultural school and the shorteners of psychoanalysis.

A. Object-Relations

In Chapter III I described how Freud's theoretical speculations during the first world war led him to elaborate a pseudo-neurological model which differed considerably from the model which he used in talking to his patients. This 'metapsychology', as he called the model, has come to provide the technical language in which orthodox Freudians now discuss their cases and theories amongst themselves; although they still find that in order to treat their patients they must talk to them in terms of memories, feelings, likes and dislikes and other familiar but non-technical concepts. Ever since the first world war, however, a small but increasing body of psychoanalysts has been developing a technical language which is not only intelligible to the patient but also reasonably suited to the technical discussion of clinical phenomena.

This development, although originally founded on a clinical observation of Freud's, began with Karl Abraham (1877–1925). From 1904 to 1907 Abraham worked under Bleuler at the Burghölzli Hospital in Zürich, and his early clinical experience was therefore with a quite different kind of patient from those who had been the subjects of Freud's trials, errors and successes. The inmates of the Burghölzli were what were then called 'dementia praecox' cases, but would nowadays be called 'psychotics', whereas Freud's hysterics, phobics and hypochondriacs were what are now called 'neurotics'. Freud thought that a psychosis was a case in which the defence-mechanisms that keep the normal person happy and allow the neurotic to maintain some sort of link with reality had proved insufficient and broken down, with the result that the unconscious, with its unrealistic phantasies and impulses, had taken over the whole mind. On this view, which is still held by many psychoanalysts, everyone can be placed somewhere on a scale, with the normal person at one end, the psychotic at the other, and the neurotic in between, and the difference between a severe neurosis and a mild psychosis is merely one of degree. Another theory is that neurosis and psychosis are two things as different in kind as tuberculosis and rheumatism:[1] on this theory a person could be either psychotic or neurotic or both or neither. Whether the difference is one of kind or degree, the symptoms and ways of thinking of psychotics do differ from those of neurotics, and both Abraham and his colleague Jung contributed new ideas to psychoanalysis which were derived in part at least from their experience of psychotic patients, although, as we have seen, Jung also drew ideas from other, non-clinical, sources.

Abraham left the Burghölzli Hospital in 1907, the year of his first meeting with Freud. He became one of Freud's inner circle, but practised psychoanalysis in Berlin, where he became the leader of the small band of German psychoanalysts. But he retained his interest in psychosis, especially in depressive states (sometimes called 'melancholia'), and his followers seem to find his ideas particularly illuminating when applied to this disorder.

[1] H. J. Eysenck, for example, argues this in *The Scientific Study of Personality* (1952), from a statistical analysis of the results of a number of kinds of test.

In his description of the super-ego Freud had pointed out how people often behave as if they had, as it were, preserved inside themselves the forbidding parental figures from which they had derived their moral standards. In a wartime essay[1] he observed how patients suffering from depressive states behaved like people who had lost something they loved, although in many cases they had not suffered any real bereavement. He explained this by saying that what they had suffered was not the loss of a real object, but the unconscious loss of an object which they had, as it were, incorporated inside themselves. Thus a woman who has ceased to love her husband (although he is still alive and with her) may exhibit all the symptoms of genuine mourning which would be appropriate if he were dead.

Abraham saw the value of this notion of incorporated objects, and proceeded to use it to explain the phenomena of depressive and other psychotic states. He was extremely interested in the stages of infantile development which preceded what Freud called the 'genital' stage—that is, in the oral phase (in which the infant seems to derive the greatest pleasure from sucking, biting and the other things which it can do with its mouth), and in the anal phase (in which the processes of excretion become exceedingly important to the child). He believed that the oral phase was responsible for the way in which the human animal behaved as if it had taken inside itself objects of which it was fond, and even objects which it hated.

Among the people to whom Dr. Abraham gave a training analysis in Berlin was Mrs. Melanie Klein, who had already studied psychoanalysis under Ferenczi in Budapest. Mrs. Klein, who began to treat children by psychoanalytic methods in 1919, came to London in 1926. As will be seen from the short history of child psychotherapy in Appendix A, she was one of the first people to attempt to treat children under six years of age on psychoanalytic principles, and to realize that in order to do so it is not sufficient to rely on verbal communication. Young children cannot, for example, carry out 'free association'. She therefore evolved the technique of 'play-analysis', in which the therapist observes the way in which the child plays with toys, and talks to the child while he is doing so; this is based on the assumption that the child's play symbolizes the difficulties he is experiencing in his relationships at home. These

[1] 'Mourning and Melancholia', 1917 (*Collected Papers*, Vol. IV).

relationships are not only with his parents (and to a lesser extent his siblings) but also with parts of his parents' bodies, and especially his mother's breast. If his experience of these objects is happy, they become 'good objects', but if it is unsatisfactory, they become 'bad objects'. Both good and bad objects are preserved in the child's unconscious memory (in technical language are 'introjected'), and colour his attitude to people and situations for the rest of his life. She found a close resemblance between the temporary reactions of a child to some event such as the loss of some loved object and the more permanent reactions which in adults are diagnosed as 'depression' or some other psychosis.

The technical language of 'object-relations' has been elaborated by Dr. W. R. D. Fairbairn of Edinburgh, who has shown, among other things, how it can be used to explain not only the marked abnormalities of psychosis (as Abraham had tried to show) but also the development of the neuroses, and how it can be used to describe the development of the ego in both normal and abnormal personalities. His technique differs only in minor ways from that of the orthodox Freudian, but he has drawn attention to an important logical point. Freud's model of unconscious ideas and forces working inside the individual is not one into which this new conception of 'object-relations' really fits. If we are going to think of behaviour as determined not only by the individual's relationships to people in the world of reality but also by the relationships with her parents which she introjected as an infant and now carries about as a world of inner object-relations, we cannot at the same time think of her behaviour as determined by the sort of inner mechanism which Freud visualized. If we are going to be logical and consistent, therefore, we must choose between the Freudian and the 'object-relations' model.

This is of course just the sort of issue in which it is important to remember what I have said in Chapter I about the use of explanatory models. Even in science it is sometimes found necessary to use two incompatible models, one for some phenomena, one for others; the 'wave' and 'quantum' models of light are examples. What is even more important is that we are dealing here with a technique and not a science, and, what is more, a technique that involves communicating with people. It is therefore less essential that the models used should be of universal utility than that they should be handy to use in the consulting-room. In other words, the best model is the one which best serves two uses. It must enable the technician to understand what his patient says, make a quick diagnosis and decide what he should reply; and it should if possible be sufficiently lifelike to enable his reply to be understood by the patient without too laborious a process of translation from technical into everyday language.

The language which most Kleinian psychoanalysts use amongst themselves is a mixture of object-relations and Freudian metapsychology, while they talk to their patients in a mixture of object-relations and the language of unconscious memories and feelings which Freud used to his patients. Orthodox Freudians, on the other hand, do not at present seem to have a terminology which is equally suitable for both technical discussion and communication with their patients. It is therefore highly probable that the object-relations terminology is in process of superseding the Freudian metapsychology as the official language of British psychoanalysis.

Technically, however, Kleinian psychoanalysts differ from orthodox neo-Freudians in only a few respects. The main differences, as Mrs. Klein herself points out,[1] were for the most part suggested by her work with children, and are as follows:

(1) *emphasis on pre-genital phases of infancy.* Mrs. Klein's experience in treating very young children has convinced her that the faulty object-relations which seem to her to lie at the root of all neurosis are formed before the child has reached the 'genital' stage of its development, and probably while it is still in the 'oral' phase. In this phase its automatic reaction to objects is to put them in its mouth, and this seems to her to explain why the neurotic should behave as if she had 'introjected' or 'incorporated' objects which have failed to satisfy her in early infancy. In treating both children and adults, therefore, the Kleinian psychoanalyst will not be satisfied with anamnesis which leads back only to the early genital phase, but will seek to reach the oral phase, whereas the more orthodox neo-Freudian would do so only if the circumstances of the case seemed to call for this.[2]

---

[1] *New Directions in Psychoanalysis*, 1955, Paper I (delivered in 1952).
[2] The principle of looking to the child's early development for the starting-point of aberration was carried even further by Otto Rank, a

(2) *The use of 'deep' interpretation.* Mrs. Klein found that a child who refused at first to respond in any way became more accessible to treatment if she began by a bold and penetrating statement about the child's secret feelings.[1] She extended this technique to the treatment of adults, and both in dream-interpretation and in interpretation generally the Kleinian analyst tends to talk in terms of very deeply buried impulses and attitudes, and to offer such interpretations without trying to prepare the patient for them. More orthodox Freudians, for example, would be content at first with a rather more superficial interpretation which the patient was just able to accept without too great distress or incredulity, and would gradually arrive at the point at which she was ready for a 'deep' interpretation. What is more, they might well, as we have seen, be satisfied with an interpretation that referred only to the early genital stages of infancy, whereas the Kleinians tend to interpret in terms of earlier stages. They believe that although the patient may at first reject a 'deep' interpretation, she will unconsciously become reconciled to it if it is true. They admit that the analyst's intuition may occasionally be wide of the mark, but do not believe that a mistaken interpretation has any effect, since it does not strike any chord in the unconscious. This aspect of the Kleinian technique is clearly a legacy of Mrs. Klein's early association with Ferenczi, whose contributions to the attempt to shorten the process of analysis are described later in this chapter; but she is not concerned with accelerating treatment so much as with ensuring that it is thorough, which in her view means that it must reach the pre-genital phases.

minor seceder who traced all anxiety-neurosis to the traumatic experience of being born. His effect on technique has not been important, although he has led some psychoanalysts to regard the anamnesis of birth as the *ne plus ultra* of their craft. Indeed there have been attempts (although not, I think, by any of the schools described in this book) to trace neurosis to antenatal experiences. As Freud found, in exploring infantile experiences it is not easy to distinguish memories from phantasies, some of which may be induced by inadvertent suggestion. Whether they are memories or phantasies, the important question is whether they have a therapeutic effect: and the evidence either way rests on a very small number of cases.

[1] See, for example, *New Directions in Psychoanalysis*, loc. cit.

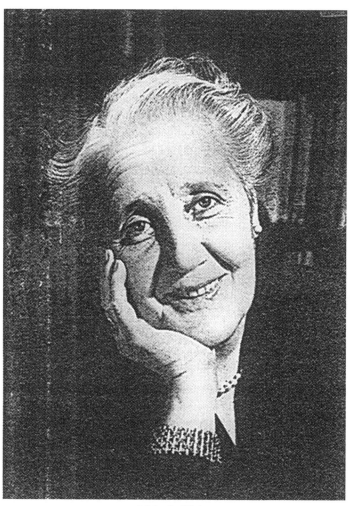

Melanie Klein.

[*to face page* 104

(3) *The emphasis on aggression and the 'death-instinct'*. Both in treatment and in theory Freud and his followers paid more attention to the libido, the affectionate side of personality, than to the aggressive instinct, which Freud probably came to recognize only under Adler's influence. This recognition seems to have taken place during the first world war, during which Freud became more and more pessimistic about human nature. At the end of the war he propounded the theory[1] that in all living organisms there operated something which was trying to restore them to their earliest state—the state of non-existence or death. This concept, which Freud called the 'death-instinct', was the product of an *a priori* piece of reasoning which is obviously fallacious. He made very little use of it in his later works, although he did try to link it up with aggression by calling the latter the 'destructive instinct', and regarding it as another form of the death-instinct which had the object of destroying not the owner but other things. He and his orthodox followers, however, made little or no use of the notion of the death-instinct in their treatment of patients.

Mrs. Klein, however, who began to treat children in Berlin in the depressing year after the armistice—the year in which Freud was writing his pessimistic essay—was struck with the extent to which aggression and even the death-instinct is observable in the very young infant. She talks of 'the vicious circle dominated by the death-instinct, in which aggression gives rise to anxiety and anxiety reinforces aggression', and says 'in the early stages of development the life-instinct has to exert its power to the utmost to maintain itself against the death-instinct'.[2] In the Kleinian treatment, therefore, of both children and adults a great deal of emphasis is laid on aggression and the death-instinct.

(4) *Attention to the transference*. The importance of the transference as a topic is of course stressed by the most orthodox of modern Freudians, but Fairbairn's object-relations model leads him to lay even more emphasis on it, and he goes so far as to refrain, like the Jungians, from insisting on the

---

[1] In *Beyond the Pleasure Principle*, 1920.
[2] *The Psychoanalysis of Children*, 1932.

patient's lying on a couch where she cannot see him; she can sit on a chair and face him if she prefers it.

(5) *Length of sessions*. Fairbairn does not adhere strictly to the Freudian session of 45 to 60 minutes, but believes that different lengths suit different patients, and is prepared to make sessions much longer if the results seem to justify it.

B. The Cultural School

Freud visited the United States in 1909 at the invitation of Stanley Hall, the President of Clark University, Massachusetts. From that date psychoanalysis gradually gained acceptance in North America, largely as a result of the efforts of A. A. Brill and Ernest Jones; and for a time its development mirrored that of orthodox Freudianism in Europe. By the middle of the nineteen-thirties, however, a movement could be distinguished that is almost distinctive enough to be called 'the American school'. I do not want to suggest that all American psychoanalysts belong to it; such uniformity would be exceptional even among psychoanalysts. Many are orthodox Freudians. But most of them stand somewhere on a scale which stretches from the Freudian point of view to that which I am about to outline.

The exodus of psychoanalysts from middle Europe which followed the rise of Nazism brought many to the United States. Among these were Mrs. Karen Horney (1885–1952), who had graduated in medicine at Berlin and had been an instructor at the Institute of Psychoanalysis there, and Erich Fromm (1900–   ), who had been a lecturer at both the Institute for Social Research and the Institute of Psychoanalysis at his birthplace in Frankfurt. They were convinced of the efficacy of Freud's therapeutic technique but questioned his theory about the nature of man's fundamental instincts and their development in the course of his growth from infancy to adulthood. Freud's experience of his nineteenth-century European patients had led him to certain conclusions which he regarded as true of any human being in any age and setting. For our purpose we can divide these conclusions into two main groups.

(A) The first group, as we saw in Chapter V, consisted of conclusions about the way in which the mind grew and worked. It includes the concepts of the ego, of repression and the other defence-mechanisms (topics which, as we saw in Chapter III, have received more and more attention in the technique of therapy), and of symbolism. These are all concepts which visualize the model as working in a particular way, and can be called the psychoanalysts' 'concepts of operation'. While the cultural school have slightly modified some of them to suit their new ideas, they have not seriously attacked them.

(B) The second group of conclusions concerned the nature of the forces which, as it were, made this mechanism tick. As we have seen, Freud thought that they were of two kinds—the sexual instincts, or libido, and the instinct of aggression (which he substituted for his early concept of the 'self-preservative instinct'). It is this group—Freud's 'motivational' conclusions—which has been seriously modified by the cultural school.

Freud thought that both these groups of instincts were part of the inborn equipment of the child. He also thought that however skilful and understanding its parents were in its upbringing these instincts must inevitably suffer a certain amount of repression and the other forms of distortion, since otherwise the child's behaviour could not be tolerated either by its parents or by society. From these and similar conclusions about innate human motives Freud came to his pessimistic conclusions about the nature of human societies. They seemed to him to be founded on the principle that the advantages of communal existence were secured at the cost of restricting man's freedom to indulge his desires, and that if man were unable to deal with his desires by repression he would be unable to live in a society.[1] In *Totem and Taboo*, for example, he argued that exogamous totem laws and the incest taboo were originally devices to prevent the family group from destroying one another in their fight over the females. In Freud's day anthropology was a very young science, and it had occurred to very few Europeans that they were not necessarily typical of all men in all cultures. There are parts of the world, for example—such as the Trobriand Islands—where infantile sexuality is not reproved, and

[1] The resemblance to Hobbes' political theory is striking. Freud had read *Leviathan* by 1914.

yet society is not disrupted (the disruption, indeed, appears to occur when Europeans try to 'civilize' such societies).

Fromm, like Adler, was a socialist and therefore more optimistic about the nature of man. His wide reading in anthropology and the history of Western Europe led him to question the universality of Freud's motivational group of conclusions, particularly those which regarded aggression as inborn. Whereas Freud had thought that the repression of aggression was the effect of society upon an inborn instinct, Fromm decided that the aggression itself, as well as the need to repress it, was the product of a particular kind of society, a society which, as a result of the breakdown of the caste-system of the Middle Ages and the opportunities offered by modern technology, encouraged ambition but at the same time had evolved an exceedingly complex system of laws and conventions which made the fulfilment of ambitions a difficult and often frustrating task. What Freud had seen as aggression and Adler as a drive for power were just as much products of this state of affairs as the repression and other distortions which had to be imposed on them if the individual was to be able to live peaceably with his family and fellow-men. Another example was the inferiority feelings which both Freud and Adler observed in their female patients; the former explained it in sexual terms as due to their consciousness of the lack of a penis, while Adler regarded it as the essence of the feminine attitude. Fromm, however, suggested that it might simply be a product of the way in which they were treated in a society in which the supply of women exceeded the demand, and pointed to cultures in which the supply-position was reversed and women were the dominant sex. In these and other ways Fromm cast doubt on Freud's notions of man's inborn drives.

The United States to which Fromm and Mrs. Horney emigrated in the early nineteen-thirties were particularly receptive to this new point of view. A large percentage of the population were either immigrants themselves or the children or grand-children of immigrants, and unlike the nationals of Western Europe they had first-hand experience of the process of adaptation to a different culture. The immigrants themselves had to undergo this process in adolescence or adulthood, and to watch their children growing up amid different social rules and values from those which had formed their own characters; while the children could see in their parents the effort to adapt at a late stage in life, and the stresses

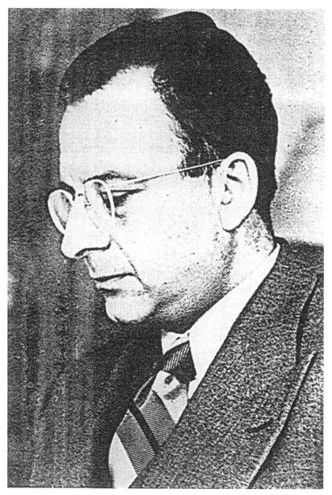

Erich Fromm.

which this caused. Geoffrey Gorer[1] has suggested that the high rate of immigration into the United States is responsible for the Americans' marked emphasis upon conformity to socially determined norms of opinion and behaviour and their suspicion of individual peculiarities. Where so many have their recent origins in an alien culture it is all-important to resemble the rest of the community as much as possible.

The practical differences in therapeutic technique that are based on this cultural point of view are differences of emphasis and terminology rather than new intermediate techniques. Fromm himself, who is primarily a sociologist, has little to say about technique, and even in the writings of the other two leaders of this school, Horney and Sullivan, the differences are implicit rather than explicit. They seem to be as follows:

(1) *Interpersonal relations.* The effects of a particular culture upon the patient are thought of in terms of her relationships to other people (and to herself), and not in terms of the ego's methods of compromising between the demands of the super-ego and id. Where a Freudian analyst would try to induce the patient to talk about the desires or fears that she feels in certain situations, and the ways in which she escapes them, the 'cultural' analyst aims at a discussion of her behaviour and feelings towards the people with whom she comes into contact. Character types are classified not in terms of the Freudian instincts (such as 'oral-sadistic') but by the way in which the person reacts to people (Horney, for example, divided patients into three groups, those who move 'towards', those who move 'against' and those who move 'away from' other people). Many patients are regarded as having built up unrealistic pictures of themselves (Horney's 'idealized image') or of other people (what Sullivan calls 'parataxic distortion') and these need to be corrected.

(2) *Anamnesis.* There is thus a tendency to deal in analysis with the patient's current experiences rather than her infantile ones. Horney even believes that patients will often talk about their infancy in order to avoid talking about their present conflicts. Not all cultural analysts go as far as this;

[1] In *The Americans,* 1947.

Sullivan, for example, still considers it useful to induce the patient to recall the circumstances in which, as a child, she began to adopt the particular attitude towards people which requires correction. But the importance of anamnesis is undoubtedly much less than in Freudian technique.

(3) *Free association.* This too is used much less, since it is valuable chiefly as a facilitant for anamnesis.

(4) *Interpretation and dream-interpretation.* The latter is still used to a considerable extent, chiefly, of course, as an indication of the patient's unconscious attitudes towards people. There is even more use of interpretation of the patient's waking thoughts and reported behaviour. It is probably true to say that the cultural analyst 'interprets' the patient's behaviour to her just as frequently and as frankly as he thinks he can do without placing too great a strain on her.

(5) *Attitude towards unconscious.* There is of course less tendency to assume that every patient is suffering from the repression of the same instincts, such as aggression. The cultural school believe, like Jung, that some of a patient's repressed tendencies are good, and should not merely be allowed expression in the analyst's room, but also be encouraged outside it. Although much less attention is paid to sexuality, and there is less tendency to interpret behaviour as the effect of repressed sexuality, cultural analysts do not entirely neglect it, since (in spite of the picture painted by the American film and novel) sexual behaviour in the United States is subject to taboos as numerous and rigid as those of Europe: the American attitude towards homosexuality, for example, is much less tolerant than the European.

(6) *Role of psychoanalyst.* There is thus a tendency for the analyst to play a much more positive role in treatment. Where the Freudian would abstain as much as possible from expressing opinions about what his patient is saying (chiefly because he is trying to avoid 'suggestion'), the cultural analyst will express approval or disapproval of certain tendencies, and will sometimes point out inconsistencies in the patient's attitudes in an almost Adlerian manner.

(7) *Self-analysis.* Dr. Horney also advocated what might be regarded as one addition to the Freudian techniques—self-

analysis.[1] While she was not the first writer, she was probably the first practising psychoanalyst to do so. Earlier
advocates of this technique, who have acquired only a
superficial knowledge of psychotherapy, have proposed it
as a substitute for psychoanalysis by a practitioner. Dr.
Horney did not altogether rule this out, but made the more
cautious suggestion that a patient who has had enough
treatment from a psychoanalyst to grasp its principles can
use this knowledge either during gaps in treatment or after
it has terminated to achieve further improvement. Not many
practising Freudians or neo-Freudians would support this
suggestion with any enthusiasm. It is true that Freud
claimed to have psychoanalysed himself for some years from
1897 onward; but he was at the same time acquiring insight
into the workings of the mind by treating other people.
What is more, he seems to have begun this analysis towards
the end of the 'primitive phase' (see Chapter II), so that by
his own later standards it was probably a fairly crude process;
certainly it did not cure or even greatly alleviate his own
psychosomatic or psychic symptoms.

C. Shortening Psychoanalysis

The greatest disadvantage of any form of psychotherapy is the
length of time for which it is necessary to treat the patient, and
this is particularly true of psychoanalysis. In its primitive phase,
when it was employed to remove the physical symptoms of hysteria,
it was a matter of weeks; in its middle phase, when it began to aim
at a wider range of symptoms and a more thorough cure, it became
a matter of years. Even today, Freud's own estimate of 'six months
to three years' (see Chapter III) would not be regarded as too
pessimistic by orthodox psychoanalysts. Most of them accept the
length of the process as an inevitable price for a reliable result;
but ever since the middle phase there have been some who have
cast about for methods of shortening it.

The first of these were Stekel and Ferenczi, two early members
of Freud's inner circle. Stekel, a Viennese physician who had
undergone a short analysis by Freud about 1901, began to practise

[1] In *Self Analysis*, 1941.

a year or two later, and claimed to be able to achieve results in 'three or four months'. Ferenczi was a Hungarian general practitioner who from 1908 until his death in 1933 was one of Freud's closest personal friends. Between them these two experimented with several modifications of technique:

(a) in some cases the analyst would, at an early stage in treatment, name a definite period beyond which he would not extend treatment; the patient was thus given, at least in theory, an incentive to rapid progress (this was probably first tried by Ferenczi);

(b) if the patient was making no headway the analyst would announce his intention of breaking off the treatment (this was probably first tried by Stekel);

(c) instead of relying on the patient's spontaneous dreams and phantasies the analyst would order the patient to enter into a phantasy about a certain situation ('forced phantasy' was probably first tried by Ferenczi, but was also used by Stekel);

(d) instead of waiting until the patient spontaneously recalled a childhood incident, or was ready to accept an interpretation of her thoughts or conduct, the analyst would force such a memory or interpretation on her, however painful and disturbing it might be ('forced interpretation' was often tried by Stekel, and, as we have seen, it is used by Kleinian analysts today, although not with the primary object of shortening treatment);

(e) the analyst would try to prevent the patient, so far as was possible, from gratifying the needs that were involved in her neurosis (this 'rule of abstinence' was probably a contribution of Ferenczi's, although we find Freud himself advocating it in a lecture of 1919). A crude example is the temporary banning of sexual satisfaction for a patient whose difficulties appear to be sexual in origin, but it is applied in much wider and subtler ways; the analyst will, for example, refrain as far as possible from removing anxiety by direct reassurance, on the theory that this would remove one of the main incentives to further progress.

The combination of these modifications is usually called 'active therapy'.

THE RETURN OF HYPNOSIS

In the nineteen-forties, nearly half a century after Freud had abandoned the use of hypnosis, psychoanalysts in the United States began to experiment with it again as a means of accelerating therapy or of dealing with cases that were particularly resistant to the normal technique. Their use of hypnosis must be distinguished very clearly from the technique of 'hypnotic suggestion', the history of which is outlined in Chapter VIII. Hypnotic suggestion uses the hypnotic state to facilitate the process of suggesting to the patient that her symptoms will disappear, whereas in the hands of the psychoanalysts hypnosis was used to assist the normal intermediate techniques. Thus anamnesis was assisted by hypnotizing the patient and telling her that she was a child of, say, five years of age again; this is technically known as 'hypnotic age-regression'. Similarly, hypnotized patients can be induced to have dreams or phantasies which can be interpreted with advantage.[1] The chief practitioners of these methods, which are collectively known as 'hypnoanalysis', have been L. R. Wolberg, J. M. Schneck and M. V. Kline in the United States, where a Society for Clinical and Experimental Hypnosis was founded in 1948.

DRUGS AS FACILITANTS

Another facilitant which has become popular since the last war is the analysis of patients while they are under the influence of drugs. One of the oldest effective techniques of non-semantic psychiatry is to send the patient to sleep for long periods. The first drug to be used was alcohol, but in the nineteenth century massive doses of opium and, later, inhalations of ether and chloroform were employed; early in this century bromides and chloral became fashionable. During the first world war barbiturates were introduced for this purpose, chiefly by Kläsi in Germany and Oberholzer in Switzerland. Although Kläsi's chief objective was still the induction of a deep sleep, he reported that it was possible and beneficial to use psychotherapy on the patient while she was

---

[1] It may be objected that these methods do not avoid 'suggestion', since without it the patient could not, for example, be induced to believe that she was a child again. There is, however, no attempt to 'suggest' to the patient that her symptoms will disappear.

drifting into this sleep. In 1930 Drs. H. D. Palmer and F. J. Braceland[1] began to use a barbiturate in the Pennsylvania Hospital, U.S.A., and found that both catharsis and suggestion could be employed with patients while they were in the drugged state. In 1936 a British doctor, J. S. Horsley, reported[2] that a light state of 'narcosis' (instead of the deep sleep at which earlier practitioners had aimed) made it possible to psychoanalyse patients, and that this method, which he called 'narcoanalysis', was both quicker and better than ordinary psychoanalysis.

In 1940 Drs. W. Sargant and E. Slater, who were treating the sudden and acute hysterias and other neuroses among the British soldiers after the retreat through Dunkirk, found that intravenous injections of barbiturates such as sodium amytal allowed the patient to recall and talk freely about the experiences that had led to the onset of his symptoms, which thereupon began to disappear. It was in this sort of case, in which the symptoms had appeared recently and suddenly after a single traumatic experience, that anamnesis facilitated by a barbiturate was most effective. Where the symptoms had appeared gradually and had persisted for some time they were more difficult to eradicate by this technique, and in some such cases Sargant and Slater employed suggestion on the drugged patients. Where more than a few sessions of this kind were required they sometimes replaced sodium amytal with hypnosis as a facilitant for anamnesis or suggestion.[3]

Various combinations of these expedients for shortening the process of treatment are now used by practitioners whose technique and theory are unmistakably Freudian, particularly in the U.S.A.[4] Many psychoanalysts, however, and especially the more orthodox British ones, are opposed to them. They argue that while hypnosis or drugs temporarily break down the barrier that separates the patient's conscious from her unconscious mind, this is done too quickly, so that the patient must either forget or in some other way dissociate herself from what she has said under the influence of the facilitant, since otherwise she would be intolerably distressed by it. Clearly this is a risk against which the users of

[1] As reported in the *American Journal of Psychiatry*, 1937.
[2] In the *Journal of Mental Science*, 1936.
[3] *An Introduction to Physical Methods of Treatment in Psychiatry*, by W. Sargant and E. Slater, 1946.
[4] A rare example of the use of a drug to facilitate Jungian treatment is recorded in Chapter VI.

hypnoanalysis or narcoanalysis must guard, and it must certainly impose a limit on the extent to which it is safe to accelerate psychotherapy by these facilitants. Even the shortening expedients of Stekel and Ferenczi are regarded with a suspicious reserve by the more orthodox psychoanalysts, on the grounds that they do not really enable the fundamental sources of the neurosis to be identified and treated.

At the same time, even the purest of Freudians are showing, I think, an increasing tendency to approach their cases in a slightly different way. Instead of asking themselves whether there is any aspect of the patient's difficulties which they have not thoroughly explored, they are more inclined to ask which are the aspects which really must be explored, and which they can afford to leave untouched. It is, for example, worth considering whether a particular patient's marital difficulties cannot be sufficiently alleviated by exploring her childhood relationship to her father, and without touching on earlier experiences connected with her mother, although these may well be partially responsible for her neurosis. In deciding a question of this sort the analyst will have in mind the fact that to embark on this further stage will probably involve many more months of treatment, which will place a further strain on the patient and may not, in the end, produce a proportionate improvement. Such a step would probably be considered justifiable only if the patient's symptoms were still severe, or if she were undergoing analysis as part of her training as a psychoanalyst. There is thus, even for the most orthodox of psychoanalysts, always the question as to the 'depth' to which it is advisable to carry the analysis, and in answering this question the time-factor is, I think, being given increasing weight.

There are thus two very different trends in mid-century psychoanalysis. In Britain, where psychoanalysts are comparatively few, closely organized and resistant to the influence of Adler, there is a tendency towards a technique that goes even deeper than orthodox Freudian practice. It traces defects of personality back to the earliest stages of infancy, and makes more use than Freud of the notions of aggression and the death-instinct. At the same time it is evolving an improved model that is taking the place of Freud's metapsychology. In the United States, on the other hand, where the process of adaptation to the codes of a new society is still going on, and the influence of Adler has been stronger, the trend is towards a more superficial technique, which lays more stress on the individual's relationship to society rather than on her early development, and therefore makes less use of anamnesis and free association. It also questions the doctrine of innate aggression and repressed sexuality. It is more anxious for quick results, and less afraid of unorthodoxy. It has thus led to the reintroduction of hypnosis, this time as a facilitant not of suggestion but of the intermediate techniques of psychoanalysis, and also—as we shall see in Chapter IX—to a readiness to experiment with new techniques such as group psychotherapy.

Recommended Reading

For British developments—

TRENDS IN PSYCHOANALYSIS, by Marjorie Brierley. Hogarth Press, 1947.
NEW DIRECTIONS IN PSYCHOANALYSIS, by M. Klein, P. Heiman, R. Money-Kyrle. Hogarth Press, 1955.

For developments in the U.S.A.—

PSYCHOANALYSIS: EVOLUTION AND DEVELOPMENT, by Clara Thompson. Allen and Unwin, 1952.
PRESENT-DAY PSYCHOLOGY, Pt. III, edited by A. A. Roback. Peter Owen, 1955.

VIII

SUGGESTION AND CONDITIONING

ALL the psychotherapeutic techniques which I have so far described are descended from Freud, whether he would have recognized them as legitimate or not. There is, however, one strain which has practically no Freudian blood in it, except occasionally by marriage. It is so loosely organized, and its rules are so much a matter of individual preference, that it is hardly a 'school' in the same sense as the Freudian or Jungian techniques; but it represents an approach to the problem which has not been altogether obliterated by the wide popularity of the Freudian and allied techniques.

THE NANCY PRACTITIONERS

In Chapter II I gave a short account of the therapeutic history of hypnotism in Western Europe up to the point at which the Freudian technique began to develop out of it. Hypnotism was studied by two schools in France—the Salpêtrière, where Charcot used it in his experiments on hysterics, and Nancy, where Freud learned from Bernheim how to make the patient repeat her anamnesis after she had emerged from the hypnotic state. The main point of difference between the two schools was that the Salpêtrière regarded the hypnotic state as itself a pathological symptom, which was confined to hysterics, while the Nancy school believed that it could be induced, to a greater or lesser degree, in normal people. We know nowadays that the Nancy school were right; the explanation of the disagreement is probably that the Salpêtrière were so interested in hysterics that they neglected to persevere with normal 'controls'. It is also possible that they paid less attention to the technique of hypnotism than the Nancy school: certainly Charcot, as we have seen, left the hypnotizing of patients to an assistant, and confined himself to demonstrating and lecturing over their bodies.

At all events it is from Nancy that modern suggestive therapy is descended. The clinic was founded in 1860 by the country doctor Liébeault (1823–1904), who obtained voluntary subjects for his hypnotic experiments by telling the avaricious French peasants, 'If I treat you with drugs I shall be compelled to charge you, but if you are treated by hypnosis I will do it for nothing.' He and his pupil Bernheim, a teacher in the Nancy medical school, achieved their cures by hypnotic suggestion. Like Freud's first patients, most of theirs seem to have suffered from marked physical symptoms, such as hysterical paralysis or the 'lassitude' that characterizes neurasthenia. Under hypnosis the patient would be told by the physician that his symptoms would disappear. With this method the school claimed success in 90 per cent of cases.

Like all successful technicians they sought for an explanation of their results. The first stage in this explanation was the observation that 'suggestion' could take place in a subject who had never been hypnotized. If they told a man that he was wearing clothes which had been worn by a sufferer from a skin disease, he would begin to itch. If a patient was told that a bottle of coloured water would relieve his cough, it would in fact alleviate it. They therefore concluded that the effect of hypnotic suggestion was merely a special instance of the effect of suggestion on human beings in general—in other words that hypnosis was merely a facilitant. Another thing which they observed was that the subjects who could be most easily hypnotized were those who responded most readily to suggestion in their normal state. Both these observations were undoubtedly valuable. There are differences between the effects of hypnotic suggestion and those of ordinary suggestion—it is easier for example to produce anaesthesia or hallucinations in the hypnotic state—but these seem to be differences of degree rather than of kind. What is more, there is no doubt that the hypnotic state itself is usually, if not always, produced by a technique which makes use of suggestion. The trick of concentrating the subject's attention on an object whose brightness and position will tire the eyes, and of lulling him with monotonous sounds or soothing music, makes him readier to accept the hypnotist's suggestion that he is having difficulty in keeping his eyes open, and is feeling drowsy. Since his eyes *are* feeling tired, and because the sounds *are* soporific, he recognizes that the hypnotist is telling the truth, and he is readier to accept his statements when he goes on to say that he cannot open his eyes without permission.

The mere description of hypnotic phenomena in terms of human suggestibility was not of course an explanation, unless of the spurious kind which I have called 'explanation by summary' (see Chapter I). To provide an explanatory model for the phenomena of suggestion in general and of hypnotic suggestion in particular the Nancy school resorted, like Freud, to the nineteenth-century conception of 'ideas'. These, as I explained in Chapter II, were thought of as solid objects, like the atoms of nineteenth-century physics, which interacted according to more or less mechanical laws. They could oust one another from consciousness, much as one billiard-ball 'pockets' another; and they produced physiological effects by operating the nervous system in some way which was never very clearly described. The stronger the emotion which was attached to them, the stronger the effect. Bernheim, and his pupil Levy, thought that the effects of suggestion were achieved by implanting in the mind of the patient an idea which would have the desired physiological effect, or which would replace one which was having an undesirable effect. A patient with hysterical paralysis of the arm was cured, they thought, because the idea of her arm as powerless to move was replaced, under suggestion, by the idea of it as a limb which she could move.

COUÉ

The member of the Nancy school who achieved the widest fame, and who was responsible for introducing its teachings to Britain and the United States, was Emile Coué (1857–1926). In the chemist's shop which he kept at Troyes, he noticed that certain drugs which he sold to his patients had beneficial effects which could not be explained physiologically, and he became convinced of the power of 'imagination'. It was only at the age of forty-four, however, that he began to study the technique of hypnotic therapy under Liébeault and Bernheim. He soon made his own modifications in both technique and theory, and nine years later, in 1910, established his own free clinic at Nancy. He was not, however, a facile writer, and produced no full-scale exposition of his views, preferring to spread them by personal lectures. It was largely his personal appearances in Britain and the United States between 1910 and his death in 1926 that aroused interest in his work, and for a written account we have to rely on his devoted disciple Baudouin (1893-   ). It is possible that most of the technical innovations were the work of Coué, and that the theoretical explanations were the contribution of Baudouin.

Coué's technical innovation seems to have been this: in the first place, he was able to use non-hypnotic suggestion to produce effects which his predecessors had found it very difficult to produce without hypnotism. Probably this was due in part to his own visible confidence in his powers; but it was also due to a trick very like that of the hypnotist. Before making any suggestion directed at the patient's symptom he would convince the patient of the power of his suggestions by making use of some physiological fact. For example, he would make her interlock the fingers of her hands, and then turn them palms outward with the arms straightened; he would then tell her that she would find it impossible to unclasp them.[1] As this is, for obvious physiological reasons, not at all easy, she would become convinced of the power of suggestion, and would in many cases be unable to unclasp her hands. After thus increasing her confidence in his powers, he would proceed to suggest that her symptoms would disappear.

Coué's best-known innovation, however, was the technique which he called 'autosuggestion'. He himself seems to have used this as a means of prolonging the effects of suggestion, which, like those of hypnotism, seemed to wear off, and had to be renewed with repetitions of the original suggestion, although at longer and longer intervals. Finally, he told his patients that they carried within themselves the means of their own cure. They could tell themselves that the ailment would disappear, and so it would; but an even better method was simply to say to themselves, just after waking and just before going to sleep, fifteen to twenty times, 'Day by day, in every way, I am getting better and better'. For, said he, 'Such general suggestion is more potent than particular suggestions'. Finally, he went a step further and recommended the use

[1] This is now the stage hypnotist's stock method of selecting from his audience the people who will make good hypnotic subjects.

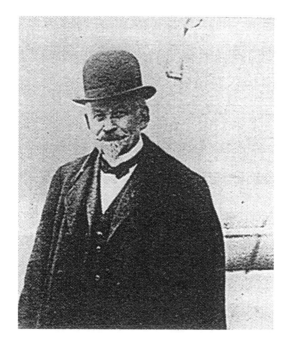

Emile Coué in his sixties.

[to face page 120

of autosuggestion without any preceding suggestion from someone else.[1]

The most ambitious claims were made for this technique. Baudouin alleged that by the combined use of suggestion and autosuggestion Coué cured such disorders as fibromata and tuberculosis (in pulmonary and other forms). The majority of the successes which he lists, however, were with disorders in which most people nowadays recognize the importance of psychological factors; examples are stammering, headaches, aphonia and certain menstrual and bowel disorders. Baudouin does not record any attempts to treat acute anxiety states, perversions or psychoses. Most of the cures are said to have taken place after one or two sessions, although one case seems to have proved resistant for some eight months.

Baudouin seems to have contributed at least one facilitant to the suggestive method. He claimed that autosuggestion was more effective if it took place while the subject was in a state which he called 'autohypnosis'. This state could be achieved by concentrating the attention either upon some external object (such as a candle-flame in a dark room) or upon some idea which was vivid enough to hold the attention without too much conscious effort; it was also helpful to have a soothing monotonous sound, such as the ticking of a clock, or to repeat aloud to oneself some short phrase which sums up the aim of the autosuggestion. The whole process was best carried out just after waking or just before going to sleep. The resemblance to some of the intermediate techniques of yoga is obvious, as Baudouin himself pointed out.

Baudouin attempted to systematize and explain the suggestive technique in his book *Suggestion and Autosuggestion*. He gives four laws of suggestion:

(1) The law of concentrated attention: 'the idea which tends to realize itself ... is always an idea on which spontaneous ATTENTION is concentrated, or an idea which has been forced on the attention after the manner of an obsession'.

(2) The law of auxiliary emotion: 'when, for one reason or another, an idea is enveloped in a powerful EMOTION, there is more likelihood that this idea will be suggestively realized'.

(3) The law of reversed effort: 'when an idea imposes itself on

[1] Compare 'autosuggestion' with 'self-analysis' (see Chapter VII).

the mind to such an extent as to give rise to a suggestion, all the conscious efforts which the subject makes in order to counteract this suggestion are not merely without the desired effect, but they actually run counter to the subject's conscious wishes and tend to intensify the suggestion'.

(4) The law of subconscious teleology: 'when the end has been suggested, the subconscious finds means for its realization'.

To explain the phenomena of suggestion, autosuggestion and hypnosis he used the ideo-motor model which had been adopted by the Nancy school. By this date, however, the model had been elaborated by the addition of what was called the 'subconscious mind'. This concept had developed out of the study of subjects with multiple personality, which had aroused such interest among French doctors and psychologists (such as Janet, Binet and Ribot) towards the end of the nineteenth century. These subjects were seen by Janet (1859–1947) as cases in which some constitutional lack of cohesiveness in the mind allowed a part of it which is normally controlled by our conscious will to operate without this control, sometimes to such an extent that normal consciousness appeared to be temporarily abolished. This part of the mind which sometimes 'took over' was called the 'subconscious', and it differed from the conscious mind chiefly in its independence of our will. Otherwise, it was capable of almost all the operations which we normally regard as conscious; it could do sums (for it sometimes did so while we were asleep), it could dictate speech (as it seemed to do in automatic writing or mediums' trances) and it could control the body even better than our consciousness. It was, in fact, a primitive personality.[1]

This enabled Baudouin to explain the phenomena of suggestion, autosuggestion and hypnosis as the result of implanting an idea not in the conscious mind but in the subconscious. Since the latter was better at controlling the body, a therapeutic idea had a better chance of achieving its aim if implanted there. This also explained

[1] The French conception of 'l'inconscient' should be clearly distinguished from the Freudian unconscious, although Janet accused Freud of plagiarism. Freud's concept, although he credited it at first with the ability to calculate, was never that of a submerged but organized personality. In this sense 'l'inconscient' is often translated as 'the subconscious', a word coined by Morton Prince, who studied multiple personality in the United States. Under the influence of Freud, however, 'l'inconscient' is increasingly used in his sense.

the law of reversed effort, for the subconscious was not only independent of the will but often reacted against it.

In England, the Oxford psychologist, William Brown (1881–1952), experimented with hypnotic suggestion at King's College Hospital in 1913, and with it cured a case of amnesia. During the first world war he used it in the casualty-clearing stations behind the trenches to treat over 700 cases of amnesia, aphonia, paralysis and other symptoms of what was then called 'shell-shock'. He soon became convinced, however, of two things. The first was that excessive use of hypnosis tended to rob patients of their ability to take their own decisions or withstand further stresses. In civilian practice therefore (he took his medical degree in 1921) he preferred suggestion and autosuggestion without hypnosis, and found them useful in cases 'in which a habitual reaction of a pathological nature has grown up in the course of time'; examples were stammering, drug addiction and bed-wetting. He found, however, that his patients were most receptive to suggestion if they were in a state of 'neuromuscular relaxation' which was assisted by deep, slow breathing, and his accounts of this state[1] sound very much as if it really was a light hypnotic trance.

His second conclusion was that most of his patients were suffering not merely from Coué's 'bad suggestion' but from a more deep-seated weakness of the personality that made them vulnerable to such suggestions. Janet had come to much the same conclusion, but had attributed the weakness to a constitutional lack of cohesion in the patient's mind, about which very little could be done. The Freudian view that the condition was acquired as a result of early experience and development offered at least a hope of ameliorating it, and Brown employed Freudian methods in addition to those of Coué, often with the same patient. This combination of the two techniques was his contribution to psychotherapy, and has had a great deal of influence on those British practitioners who are not too firmly bound to Freudian or Jungian beliefs to use suggestion.

Coué's personal visits to Britain and the United States after the first world war won him some followers, who set up Institutes

---

[1] In the *British Journal of Psychology* for 1938. A letter which he wrote to the *Lancet* in February 1951 shows that by then he had come to regard the state of 'neuromuscular relaxation' as beneficial by itself, without any accompanying therapeutic suggestion. If so, he must be credited with a new intermediate technique.

in his name in London and New York. But purely suggestive methods soon lost ground to psychoanalysis outside France. They were regarded as treating symptoms rather than causes, and even so, as Coué himself admitted, their results were sometimes short-lived. Even his follower Baudouin, now at Geneva University, gradually transferred his interest to psychoanalysis.

THE IMPLICATIONS OF BEHAVIOURISM

Meanwhile the ideo-motor theory which the Nancy school used as an explanatory model had been strongly attacked by the behaviourist psychologists, particularly the American, Thorndike. Behaviourism is essentially an attempt to reduce the science of psychology to purely descriptive statements in terms of values that can be measured in the laboratory, and to do without explanatory references to 'the mind' or to any of the pheneomena of introspection. A great deal of the work of the early behaviourists was concerned with the study of animals, who cannot be asked to introspect and report the results. If you want to know whether a dog is afraid the only facts you have are its behaviour, which in the laboratory can of course include the accurate measurement of such physiological factors as its pulse-rate. This led to the description of human emotions, desires, memories and so on, in terms of physiological changes; changes in pulse-rate, activation of nerves in the central and peripheral nervous system, the secretion of adrenalin and other hormones, formed the only explanatory model which the behaviourists allowed themselves to use; they wanted to eliminate anything that could not be detected and measured by an observer.

The ideas which were regarded by the suggestive school as the instruments by which they achieved their results were introspectible things, and could not be observed in the way upon which the behaviourists insisted; they were therefore suspect. In any case they were not a very accurate way of describing even what can be observed by introspection. Most of the actions which we regard as conscious and not in the least inadvertent are not preceded or accompanied by any clear picture of what we want to do or are doing; we simply do them and 'pay attention to what we are doing'. Even when we do plan something beforehand, and arrive by a sort of trial-and-error process at a clear plan of what we are going to do, this plan does not usually consist of one idea, or even of a chain of ideas, so much as of a smooth thought-sequence. This can be chopped up into a series of separate ideas by the same sort of arbitrary division as that by which we split the day into morning, afternoon, evening, dusk and night; but to regard each of these ideas as the cause of some part of our planned action is carrying artificiality too far. Without begging any metaphysical questions, thinking is something that we do, not an infinite number of nouns which we carry about inside our heads.[1]

Behaviourism proper, however, did not have a direct effect upon therapeutic technique; it merely cast suspicion upon the intro- spective model of 'ideas', without providing any precise descrip- tion in its own language of the way in which behaviour disorders arose. But Pavlov's work on conditioned reflexes had a more direct bearing on psychiatry.

Pavlov (1849–1936) was a St. Petersburg physician, who at the age of forty-one became Professor of Pharmacology and Director of Physiology in that city's Institute of Experimental Medicine. After some physiological research on gastric juices, he began a laboratory study of a particular sector of animal behaviour. In ordinary life, the way in which a given animal (even a human being) will react to a given set of circumstances is not certain. If I say 'Rats' to a terrier, he may do one of three things: he may jump up and begin to sniff around; he may merely wag his tail; if he has never heard the word before, or if the joke is too stale, he may pay no attention. The most that can be said about this sort of behaviour is that there are a limited number of possible reactions. There are some, however, that are predictable with much more certainty. If something touches or threatens to touch my eyeball, I cannot help blinking; if something hot or sharp is pressed against my hand I jerk it away. These are called 'reflex actions', and it is this difference between them and the rest of the complex behaviour of animals that made them an attractive subject of laboratory study. The fact

[1] It is interesting, however, to note that in his description of his experi- ments with suggestibility, Eysenck says that he finds the ideo-motor terminology the most suitable to describe the way in which a subject who is made to think of some action cannot help minute movements of the muscles involved in that action. (*Dimensions of Personality*, 1947.) Some behaviourists would of course retort that it is better still to regard these muscle-movements as the important part of the process of thinking about the action.

that a given set of circumstances (called the 'stimulus') will almost invariably be accompanied by a certain action on the animal's part (called the 'response') means that the scientist can experiment to see whether there are certain conditions (such as extreme fatigue) under which this stimulus-response invariance will break down, or will alter in some way.

This is what Pavlov began to do, using for his purpose an animal that was readily available and large enough to be easily operated on—the dog (it was probably only a coincidence that it is also one of the most easily trained of animals). But instead of selecting for his study one of the usual 'stimulus-response' combinations, such as limb-withdrawal, he remained true to his interest in digestive secretions, and chose to study the salivary response that occurs when an animal is offered food. The choice was important because responses such as limb-withdrawal do not depend upon the brain, but can be produced even if the spinal cord between the limb and the brain is severed; whereas the secretion of saliva and other digestive juices is not independent of the brain. Pavlov proceeded, however, to study the salivation response in dogs as if it were a simple spinal reflex, and the result was extremely interesting.

The salivation response to the sight or smell of food occurred without any training or preparation of the animal, and he therefore classified this as an 'absolute' reflex. He found, however, that if the food is accompanied by the ringing of a bell, the ringing of this bell will eventually produce the salivation response without the offer of food. Because this reflex was the result of 'conditioning' he distinguished it from the absolute reflex by calling it 'conditioned'. Even painful stimuli such as electric shocks could, by conditioning, be made to result in the salivation response. He also observed that both absolute and conditioned reflexes could be 'inhibited', if the sight of food or the sound of the bell occurred regularly without the animal receiving the food, the salivation response disappeared.

The accidental flooding of his laboratory in 1924, and the curious disturbances which this produced in the absolute and conditioned reflexes of his experimental dogs, drew Pavlov's attention to the possibility of describing the formation and symptoms of neurosis in his terminology. He found that he could produce abnormal behaviour in three ways. He could make the stimulus (such as an electric shock or a noise) an extremely strong one. Or he could force the animal to inhibit its response for a long time or in circumstances which make this inhibition difficult (a hungry dog, for example, can be made to wait for its food for a long time after the conditioned stimulus of the ringing of the bell). Thirdly, a conflict between reflexes can be produced; a dog that has been conditioned to salivate at the sight of a luminous circle, but not at the sight of an ellipse, will exhibit abnormal behaviour when the ellipse becomes so close in shape to the circle that it has difficulty in distinguishing between the two kinds of stimuli.

These three methods, however, did not each produce a specific kind of abnormal behaviour in all the experimental subjects. Some dogs could stand stronger stimuli than others without breaking down; others could stand more inhibition. What was more interesting was that some broke down in an excitable way, and barked, bit and ran aimlessly about; while others refused to respond in any way to any of the normal stimuli. Pavlov had come to the conclusion that there were fundamentally two ways in which the neurons of the brain interacted with each other. One way was 'excitation', and the other was 'inhibition'. He therefore decided that there were two kinds of dog—the 'excitatory' and the 'inhibited'. In the excitatory dog the inhibitory neurons were outnumbered or in some other way dominated by the excitatory ones, and in the inhibited dogs the opposite was the case. In many cases the balance was fairly even, and the dog was a stable 'excitatory' or 'inhibited' type; but in extreme cases the experimental stress of over-excitation, over-inhibition or conflict led to an almost complete failure of the subordinate activity, whether it was inhibition or excitation. An excitatory dog therefore became quite unable to inhibit its reactions, while an inhibited one became unable to do anything else.

PAVLOV AND MODERN TECHNIQUES

In Western Europe Pavlov's experiments had little immediate influence upon the treatment of the neuroses. This was partly due to the popularity of psychoanalysis in one form or another at this time (the late nineteen-twenties and thirties). Another reason, however, was that he himself offered very little in the way of practical technical advice on the treatment of neuroses by semantic methods. His prescription for over-excitation was bromide, on the theory that it strengthened the inhibitory neurons; while for over-inhibition he prescribed rest, in order to recruit the excitatory cells. His influence upon Russian psychiatry, on the other hand, has been very great. After a brief period between the two world wars when psychoanalysis was practised in the Soviet Union, it is now strongly discouraged. Joseph Wortis' book *Soviet Psychiatry*, 1951, contains this summary:

> The chief features of Soviet psychotherapy at present are the following:
>
> (1) A direct appeal to rational consciousness by means of logic, persuasion, scientific enlightenment, group pressures and the creation of positive incentives. Much of this is done by preference in a group setting, and it is recognized that many educational and other agencies outside the scope of psychiatry may fulfil this function. But it is also felt that rational persuasion, unsupported by other agents, can also become too abstract and intellectual.
>
> (2) The implication and relief of physiological factors which may support tendencies to persistent obsessive ideas (Pavlov's concept of pathological inertia), depressive emotional tone, excessively frightened reactions, loss of control (i.e. weakness of inhibition), unstable moods, etc.
>
> (3) The reinforcement of positive influences through suggestion, at times by the use of hypnosis.
>
> (4) The positive removal of the patient from harmful influences, and the deliberate involvement of the patient in wholesome experience and activities, especially work activities, with the provision for the patient of the material means, equipment, proper setting and other help necessary for this purpose.

It is clear that the inspiration of Soviet psychotherapy is Pavlov's behaviouristic or reflexological outlook. Its emphasis on observable responses to the patient's present environment contrasts strongly with the importance which Freudians attach to the effects of infancy; the only concession which it makes to this point of view is in the education of the child, whose 'whole emotional equipment must be directed toward love of creation, work, collective life'.[1] There is an equally marked divergence between the Soviet

[1] Wortis, loc. cit. (reproduced by courtesy of the William Wilkins Company, of Baltimore, U.S.A.).

psychotherapist's use of the direct appeal to rational consciousness, combined with suggestion, and the Freudian attention to unconscious factors and studied avoidance of suggestion in any form.

But if Pavlov's direct influence on Western psychotherapeutic techniques between the wars was small, his effect upon scientific theory was not. Both behaviourist psychologists and experimental neurologists were encouraged to use his concepts in their study of human behaviour and the central nervous system. His ideas even reached the popular mind, so that mothers and nurse-maids attributed childish tantrums to 'over-excitement', and chaste maidens were called 'inhibited' by disappointed suitors.

One of the effects of this development was an attempt to describe the phenomena of psychotherapy, and particularly psychoanalysis, in behaviourist or reflexological terms. In 1936 Professor John Macmurray suggested[1] that the behaviourists' language of 'habit' and 'learning' could be used in this way. He pointed out that very few of our responses to events are uncontrollable reactions; most of them are acquired by conscious learning. We learn to eat, talk and walk by what are at first conscious efforts but soon become unconscious automatisms. If we learn some incorrect way of talking or walking and want to put it right we can do so only by making the action conscious and deliberate again and then relearning it the right way. Macmurray suggested that what was troubling the psychotherapists' patients was some reaction, once fully conscious but now automatic and uncontrollable, that was interfering with normal behaviour. Thus the therapeutic process of psychotherapy consisted of making the incorrect reaction conscious in order to let it be relearnt in the right form.

In 1941 Dr. Roland Dalbiez showed how Pavlov's reflexological language could be used to describe phenomena to which Freud had drawn attention. Pavlov himself had of course asserted that the neuroses which he induced in his dogs and those which could be observed in human beings were of the same nature, but he had not attempted a detailed exposition of this point of view. Dalbiez, for example, compared the conflict-neurosis in the dog that could not distinguish between the circle-stimulus and the ellipse-stimulus with the neurosis which Freud had observed in what he called the 'Oedipus-situation'. It is not uncommon for men who in boyhood

[1] In the Deems Lectures, eventually published as *The Boundaries of Science*, 1939.

were abnormally attached to their mothers (for example, the only sons of widows) to suffer from impotence or other sexual difficulties. Dalbiez argued that

> the fundamental difficulty of the Oedipus-situation consists in this, that a certain complex stimulus [the mother] ought not to arouse the genital reaction, whereas another complex stimulus closely resembling the former [another woman] ought to arouse it. Thus formulated, the difficulty of the Oedipus-situation is merely a sexual instance of the clash between excitation and inhibition by differentiation. . . .[1]

In a similar way Dalbiez described other Freudian observations in Pavlovian terms.

It will be clear from what I have said in Chapter I that these are not rival explanations to the Freudian model. They merely assert that the phenomena observed by Freud are instances of a very large class of phenomena which have been studied in the laboratory. This does not explain the phenomena any more than you explain the increasing length of a bar of iron in the sun by saying that it is an instance of the expansion of metal under heat. Nor is it of any technical assistance to the psychotherapist, since it does not suggest to him any improvement in his methods.[2] But it is not altogether beside the point. The fact that it is possible to describe the observations of psychotherapists in the language of 'learning theory' or 'reflexology' seems to justify psychotherapists in paying attention to the individual's past experiences and present feelings, rather than to the possibility of defect, inherited or acquired, in the individual's nervous system, although it does not of course rule out the theoretical possibility of a neurological explanation of this kind. Moreover, Macmurray's 'habit-relearning theory' (as I call it) is very relevant to two points that worry psychotherapists. These are the slowness of the therapeutic process and the fact that this slowness increases with the age of the patient.

---

[1] *Psychoanalytic Method and the Doctrine of Freud* (tr. Lindsay), 1941, Vol. II.

[2] Indeed it is noticeable that Dalbiez offers some very plausible accounts in Pavlovian terms of the neuroses observed by Freud, but does not offer any Pavlovian description of the process of cure or alleviation. This is attempted, however, by Professor Macmurray, and, in more detailed and technical language, by psychologists such as Dr. O. H. Mowrer (for example, in a paper on 'Progress in Clinical Psychology' (ed. Brower and Abt), 1952).

Are these due to defective technique? Probably not, if Macmurray is right in classifying psychotherapy as a phenomenon of learning. We all know what long practice it takes to relearn a faulty habit, even a comparatively superficial one like a golf-swing; and we all know that as we grow older we find it harder to learn new tricks or unlearn old ones.

Since the second world war, however, reflexology and behaviourism have had slightly more influence on psychotherapy outside the U.S.S.R. One example is the method devised by Dr. O. H. Mowrer in the U.S.A. for the treatment of bed-wetting (or 'enuresis'). This is a common disorder among children deprived of normal parental care or affection, and is usually treated by drugs, psychotherapy or retribution. Mowrer invented a simple apparatus which awoke the child by ringing a bell as soon as it began to wet the bed; and he claimed that this rapidly cured the disorder without replacing it with any other symptoms. Another example is what is called 'aversion therapy', quite frequently used to treat addictions to alcohol or tobacco, and more rarely in cases of other disorders.[1] The essence of this method is to arrange, usually by administering a drug such as apomorphine, that the patient will feel nauseated when drinking alcohol, smoking a cigarette or doing whatever he wants to stop doing. After this has been carried out several times, the patient feels nauseated by the stimulus without any artificial assistance.[2]

A third example is the attempt of Andrew Salter in the U.S.A. to use Pavlovian theory as a basis for a technique of hypnotic and non-hypnotic suggestion that is strongly reminiscent of Coué. The reflexologist regards words as 'conditioned stimuli'. Just as it is possible, by associating the presence of food with the ringing of a bell, to make the dog salivate at the sound of the bell when food is no longer offered, so the constant uttering of the word 'food' to a man who is being offered food will eventually turn the word by itself into a 'conditioned stimulus' that will produce the response

---

[1] See, for example, a report on 'A Case of Fetichism Treated by Aversion Therapy', by Dr. M. J. Raymond, in the *British Medical Journal*, 1956.

[2] It is a nice question whether this should be regarded as a semantic or as a non-semantic sub-technique. But it seems to me to differ from other kinds of treatment by drugs because in this case the drug is merely a convenient method of conditioning the patient to respond in a certain way to a certain stimulus.

appropriate to food. This explains why almost every human being, having been conditioned to a large number of verbal stimuli in childhood, can be made to respond with physiological changes to words. When a man is made to shiver by being told that the room is cold, he is responding to the conditioned stimulus without the presence of the unconditioned one. 'Suggestion' is therefore nothing more than the use of words as conditioned stimuli in a more extreme and spectacular way than usual; and hypnosis is a state in which this is particularly easy (Pavlov regarded it as a state of inhibition of the more complex responses which would normally prevent the subject from responding in quite such a simple way).

Salter describes[1] how he uses his technique to treat most forms of neurosis—phobias, addictions, insomnia, sexual aberrations and some psychosomatic symptoms. He believes that these disorders occur in what he calls 'inhibitory personalities' who are prevented by their 'conditioning' from reacting to stimuli with the appropriate emotions and actions. Part of his technique therefore consists of encouraging his patients to become what he calls 'excitatory', and to respond emotionally to everyday events instead of remaining impassive. The rest of his technique is recognizably that of Nancy. A patient who complains of insomnia, for example, is conditioned in the consulting-room, by hypnotic or non-hypnotic suggestion, to feel drowsy when Salter snaps his fingers (or provides some other easily reproduced stimulus): eventually the patient is enabled to make herself feel drowsy by snapping her own fingers, and may even be able to produce this effect by imagining the sound. Like Coué he uses anamnesis only to discover the nature of the original 'bad suggestion', although he himself would call it 'faulty conditioning'.

Salter is interesting because his technique, so obviously descended from Coué's, is no longer based on the nineteenth-century ideo-motor model but draws its technical language from twentieth-century reflexology. It is still possible, however, to find a few preachers of pure Couéism, both in technique and in theory. A book published in 1950[2] by the stage hypnotist, Ralph Slater, contains a chapter on the treatment of smoking, alcoholism, stuttering, frigidity, impotence and homosexuality by the technique of

[1] *Conditioned Reflex Therapy*, 1949.
[2] *Hypnosis and Self-Hypnosis*, 1950.

hypnotic suggestion, reinforced by autosuggestion; the theoretical explanations might have been written by Coué himself.

In Britain there is a small Society of Medical Hypnotists which, unlike its counterpart in the U.S.A. (see Chapter VII), is more interested in hypnotism as a facilitant for suggestion than as a facilitant for the intermediate techniques of psychoanalysis. Its President, Dr. S. J. Van Pelt, advocates hypnotic suggestion in the treatment of neurasthenia; anxiety states; hysteria; obsessional neurosis; depression; the 'nervous element' in such organic disorders as angina pectoris or high blood pressure, pain in incurable disease; 'bad habits' such as alcoholism, sexual perversions or bed-wetting; 'painful and obscure conditions' such as migraine, trigeminal neuralgia or phantom limb; and skin conditions such as neurodermatitis, rosacea, eczema, urticaria and psoriasis.

Quite apart from its psychotherapeutic use, hypnotic suggestion is now being employed analgesically. Physical methods of abolishing severe pain, whether in dentistry, childbirth or surgery, have their disadvantages; some require an elaborate technique for safe administration, and some have unpleasant side-effects on the patient, particularly if she is weak or elderly. Hypnotic suggestion is therefore increasing in popularity as an analgesic, particularly in dentistry and obstetrics.

The attraction of suggestion or conditioning as psychotherapeutic sub-techniques lies of course in the fact that where they achieve results these are rapid and spectacular. Some practitioners of other kinds of psychotherapy are ready to make use of these methods in certain cases (as William Brown was), but most believe that the effects are temporary and confined to the symptom of which the patient complains, so that character-disorders of which the patient may not be aware are left untreated. The second of these criticisms is obviously true, and the first is probably true of certain disorders or patients. But until other psychotherapeutic schools have succeeded in accelerating the process of cure and in dealing with all the varieties of psychogenic disorder, they can hardly afford to neglect these methods entirely.

Recommended Reading

LA PSYCHOLOGIE CONTEMPORAINE, by P. Foulquié and G. Deledalle, pp. 215–19. Presses Universitaires de France, 1951.

SUGGESTION AND CONDITIONING

SUGGESTION AND AUTOSUGGESTION, by C. Baudouin. Allen and
Unwin, 1920.

SUGGESTION AND MENTAL ANALYSIS, by William Brown, 1922.

SOVIET PSYCHIATRY, by Joseph Wortis. William and Wilkins, 1950.

CONDITIONED REFLEX THERAPY, by Andrew Salter. Allen and Unwin,
1952.

THE BRITISH JOURNAL OF MEDICAL HYPNOTISM.

IX

GROUP PSYCHOTHERAPY

MOST of the techniques which I have outlined in this book have been based on the assumption that their effects could best be achieved in confidential, tête-à-tête conversations between patient and therapist. This assumption arose naturally from Freud's original theory that the therapeutic process worked in a cathartic way, and that the patient grew better through purging herself of secret thoughts and memories. If this were so, it seemed to follow that she would unburden herself more readily and thoroughly if she were talking in complete confidence and privacy to one person. Although the inadequacies of the cathartic theory were fairly soon recognized by psychoanalysts, including Freud himself,[1] several assumptions based on it have survived, and this is one of them. The typical psychotherapeutic interview is still carried on in complete privacy. Since even the treatment of the mildest disorders by the most superficial psychotherapeutic technique requires numerous and frequent interviews, each between half an hour and an hour in length, the result is that very few patients can be treated at any one time by a single psychotherapist. Twelve sessions a day on five and a half days a week are the practical limit for any normal psychotherapist, and even this places quite a strain on him. If he sees the average patient three times a week this will allow him to have not more than twenty-two under treatment at any one time. This doctor-patient ratio of 1 : 22 is very much lower than in any other field of medicine, and is of course the reason why psychotherapeutic treatment is so expensive. As a result, institutions which have to cope with large quantities of neurotic or psychotic patients—such as State or Military hospitals—are taking an increasing interest in the

[1] See Chapter III.

possibility of treating more than one patient in the same psychotherapeutic interview; that is, in group psychotherapy. This interest is not confined to one particular school; group psychotherapy is practised by therapists from almost all the sects which we have been considering, and as we shall see its effects are interpreted by each in the light of their own theories.[1]

SUGGESTION AND GROUPS

Suggestive forms of psychotherapy have been practised on groups of people ever since they began to be used. Mesmer treated his patients in groups. Coué's sessions at Nancy were group-sessions; according to Baudouin, he would treat about thirty patients at one time, with another thirty waiting their turn in the garden outside. This may have been due simply to his desire to treat as many people as possible; we know that he did treat some of his famous patients in private sessions, although this may have been at their desire. I suspect, however, that Coué had discovered not merely that numbers were no obstacle but also that he could achieve his effects more quickly and easily in a group.

DIDACTIC GROUPS

Quite independently, however, doctors in the United States were beginning to make use of the psychological properties of groups as an aid to therapy. The first attempts were made with physical disorders. In 1905, a Dr. Pratt, who was treating tuberculous out-patients in the Boston Dispensary, began to hold classes in personal hygiene for these patients, and found that he achieved not only this practical educational aim but also a very considerable raising of their morale, which appeared to him to contribute to their recovery. Pratt, and his followers at the Dispensary, extended this method to other chronic disorders—diabetics, cardiacs, postpartum cases, women with vaginitis, sufferers from essential hypertension, people with peptic ulcers—some of which would now be recognized as having a psychological element

---

[1] This may be the reason for the extraordinary variations between different accounts of the development of group psychotherapy. For example, J. W. Klapman's book *Group Psychotherapy: Theory and Practice* (1946) contains a historical chapter which completely ignores Adlerian work in this field.

in their causation. His purely educational classes developed into frankly therapeutic sessions, which began with exercises in relaxation, and resembled Coué's sessions in this and other ways. They came to be known as 'thought-control' clinics.

By the time of the first world war two other United States doctors were beginning to use the group method in the treatment not of physical but of psychic symptoms. In a Washington Hospital Dr. E. W. Lazell found that psychotic patients—including many who were apparently inaccessible to individual treatment by psychotherapeutic methods—improved considerably if groups of them were given lectures in simplified language on psychoanalysis. About the same time Dr. L. C. Marsh was treating psychotics by group methods, first in a New York hospital and later in the Worcester State Hospital. He had noticed how mass meetings of religious revivalists achieved much more intense effects upon the audience than tête-à-tête exhortation, and he thought that the mere fact that his patients were doing something together had a beneficial effect upon them. Like Lazell, he gave lectures, but unlike him he did not think that they need be on psychiatric subjects; a talk on Russia, on how to bring up babies, or on current events, was equally therapeutic, although it was also useful for the patients to receive a simple explanation of their condition, either from lectures or from books. He also supplemented his lectures by other group activities, such as community singing and formation of committees among the patients to look after some aspect of their activities.

A modern descendant of Lazell's method is the 'didactic group therapy' of Dr. J. W. Klapman, of the Northwestern University Medical School in the United States. Like Lazell and Marsh he is dealing for the most part with psychotics in hospitals. He uses easily understood texts and lectures about mental illness and its causes; sessions at which case-histories are read out to an audience of patients; other types of session at which each patient writes his own autobiography; discussions on psychotherapeutic subjects; and discussions on any subject likely to interest the group.

PSYCHODRAMA

Another technique was developed in Vienna just after the first world war by Dr. J. L. Moreno (1892–   ). As a medical student he had become interested in the possibilities of what he called the Theatre of Spontaneity (*Stegreiftheater*). Instead of using professional actors to play rehearsed parts he would induce volunteers from his audiences to enact scenes prompted by their own 'private worlds'. Although his early experiments on these lines were part of the attempts in post-war Russia and Germany to free the theatre from its traditional formalism, he soon began to see that an actor whose scenes portrayed 'his private world, his personal problem, his own conflicts, defeats and dreams' was achieving an emotional catharsis, and that the technique thus had therapeutic possibilities. It was particularly useful for patients who could not form a transference to a therapist. As examples of these he cited children and psychotics, although few psychotherapists would agree nowadays that children do not form a transference, and even psychotics may do so in certain circumstances. After using this technique in private practice in Vienna, Moreno migrated to the United States in 1927, and in 1936 founded a Sanitarium where he practised it.

The theatre which he designed for this purpose is small. The stage consists of three concentric circular aprons, rising in broad steps from the audience's seats. It has a balcony overhead which can be used in the drama, but where the psychotherapist usually sits. He acts as producer, and has male and female assistants who are ready to play parts in the drama. His talks with the patient have indicated to him the sort of scene which should be played; it may portray some actual event from her past, but is more often the expression of phantasy. It may involve her parents, her friends, or even, in the case of psychotic patients, the devil or other imaginary being who prompts or torments them; all these parts are usually played by the psychotherapist's assistants. Other patients usually form the audience, who are encouraged to discuss and even participate, emotionally and physically, in the action. As far as possible, however, the nature of the action is determined by the patient herself, although she may need a good deal of active prompting from producer and assistants, particularly at first.

Although Moreno dissociates himself firmly from psychoanalysis, his terminology owes a great deal to Freud and Adler. The assistants who act the parts in the patient's drama are called 'auxiliary egos', and he also talks of 'projection', 'resistance', 'reality-testing' and (an Adlerian term) the patient's 'life-line'. In essence his theory is a very simple combination of the early

Freudian notion of catharsis and the Adlerian notion of 'community-feeling'. Aristotle pointed out the cathartic effect of drama upon the audience; Moreno insists that its cathartic effect upon the actor is even greater.[1] He also insists that as a means of inducing the emotions of which the patient is to be purged, acting is superior to talking; the stage is mightier than the consulting-room. He also believes that acting in the presence of an audience, who are encouraged to comment freely and even to take part in the drama, helps to bring the patient into closer touch with the society in which he ought to be able to live comfortably.

ADLER'S GROUPS

Adler's contribution to group psychotherapy seems to have begun with his child guidance clinics, of which the first was set up in Vienna in 1921. His procedure was to interview the child, either with or after its parents, in the presence of other parents, children and teachers. One of his motives was undoubtedly to spread an understanding of his methods, but he also argued that there was positive justification for it:

> The public character of these clinics has often been attacked. Our experience has shown, however, that the appearance of the child before a large gathering has a stimulating effect upon him. The publicity of the procedure suggests to the child that his trouble is not a private affair, since strangers are also interested in it. His social-mindedness is more awakened through this.[2]

Adler's technique of group psychotherapy was therefore really a public session with one individual. (A similar approach was used from 1936 onwards by the neo-Freudian Louis Wender in the U.S.A., who would psychoanalyse one patient in the presence of others.) On the other hand, a Viennese follower of Adler, Dr. R. Dreikurs, experimented as early as 1929 with group treatment of adult private patients as a supplement to individual sessions. It was Dreikurs, too, who seems to have been the first to experiment (in

---

[1] In both cases the drama must of course bear a close relation to a problem or difficulty in which the audience or actor are personally involved.

[2] Quoted by L. Way in *Alfred Adler*, 1956, from R. Seidler and L. Zilahi, in *Guiding the Child*.

the United States after the second world war) with what he called 'multiple psychotherapy'. In this technique, which was suggested to him by Adler's clinics and by the experience of Dr. G. Reeve in a Cleveland Mental Hospital in the nineteen-thirties, the patient is interviewed at first by a single psychotherapist, until her original reticence is overcome; she can then be treated simultaneously by two therapists. Dreikurs claims that this is a valuable adjunct to 'single' psychotherapy, and in particular that it enables the patient to be observed and treated in a wider variety of relationships.

THERAPEUTIC COMMUNITIES

Another follower of Adler, Dr. J. Bierer, saw the value of Marsh's observations of the beneficial effects of communal activity on hospital patients, and at the beginning of the second world war began to treat in-patients and out-patients at the Runwell Hospital and elsewhere in England by a combination of social activities and individual psychotherapy. Out-patient clinics on these lines are now run under his supervision at one or two London hospitals, where patients not only receive individual psychotherapy but are kept occupied in communal activities for the whole of the working day. Bierer's idea that hospitals and clinics for psychosis and neurosis could be made into 'therapeutic communities' has had considerable influence on the administration of mental hospitals in Britain. Although the idea has been interpreted in many different ways, its essential point seems to lie in ensuring that not only the psychotherapist but all the other staff are informed about the circumstances and difficulties of each patient, and are trained to treat her not only with tolerance but also with understanding. Patients are encouraged to work out any necessary rules and instructions by agreement amongst themselves, instead of having them imposed by authority; and communal activities are encouraged.

PLAY GROUPS

In 1934 S. R. Slavson (1891–) began to use a new technique in dealing with 'problem' children under the auspices of the Jewish Board of Guardians in New York. Groups of children were allowed to play freely together under the charge of the psychotherapist, who interfered as little as possible. Slavson found that the children's behaviour not only enabled him to see very clearly what each child's difficulty was, but also led to a gradual improvement in the child's symptoms; he thus distinguished clearly the diagnostic and the therapeutic uses of group treatment. Out of these 'play groups'[1] developed other kinds. Older children's groups could gradually be introduced into outside organizations—such as clubs for boys or girls—in which the children eventually took their place as normal members; these were called 'transitional groups'. Some children were either too aggressive or too frightened of other children to be allowed to become members of 'play groups'; they were formed into groups in which the therapist exercised more control over activity, and ensured that the more violent feelings of the children were expressed in talking rather than action; these were called 'activity-interview' groups. Finally, as Slavson and his followers came to deal with adolescents and adults, groups were formed in which action was replaced entirely by talk; these were called 'interview groups'.

INTERVIEW GROUPS

The second world war provided very favourable conditions for the spread of group psychotherapy. The war-time decrease in civilian neurosis was counterbalanced by its high incidence amongst servicemen. Many British psychotherapists were working in military hospitals, but needed some means of dealing with larger numbers of cases than could be handled in private interviews. Early in the war, therefore, they began to copy the group techniques which had been developed in the United States, and in particular the technique of interview groups.[2] The work at Northfield Military Hospital, which S. H. Foulkes has described,[3] was probably the largest in scale; it was practitioners such as Foulkes who saw in it not merely a *pis aller* but a technique which in some cases might achieve quicker and better results than that of private interview alone, and who therefore introduced it into private practice and civilian clinics in post-war Britain.

[1] In which Slavson sometimes used Moreno's psychodramatic technique.

[2] Although I have also found accounts of didactic group therapy on Klapman's lines, for example, by Major D. Blair, R.A.M.C., in the *Lancet* for 13th February, 1943.

[3] In *Introduction to Group Analytic Psychotherapy*, 1949.

It is the 'interview group'[1] therefore that has become the main sub-technique of modern group psychotherapy. Broadly speaking, it consists of regular meetings of the same group of patients under the guidance of the same psychotherapist, at which the patients are encouraged to talk to each other about their symptoms and eventually their personal difficulties and emotional conflicts. The extent to which the psychotherapist guides the discussions varies very greatly; Dr. W. McCann, for example, goes so far as to leave groups unsupervised in the consulting-room. The psychotherapist's practice in this matter obviously depends partly on his views as to the nature and aims of the therapeutic process, and partly, of course, on the way in which each particular group develops. In all such groups, however, the members develop and express various emotions towards each other and the psychotherapist; they also acquire in varying degrees the ability to understand and accept the emotional reactions of the other members and themselves.

Some psychotherapists use the group method to the virtual exclusion of private sessions. The most common practice, however, is to give each patient private interviews, either to prepare her for her introduction into a group or to supplement group treatment by allowing her to discuss certain matters with the psychotherapist alone. Some psychotherapists consider certain types of patient unsuitable for group treatment. Some form their groups by selecting all the patients with the same type of symptom (although in the case of some symptoms, such as homosexuality, this must obviously be avoided). Some mix the sexes in their groups, others believe that this inhibits discussion. Most keep their sessions to the same length as private interviews—that is, between 45 and 60 minutes.

There is obviously much less scope in such sessions for intermediate techniques such as anamnesis of childhood experiences, or dream-interpretation. Patients do, however, indulge in a certain amount of cathartic expression of feelings and desires which they would otherwise have kept to themselves; and in many cases the relationship with other group members seems to produce the very emotions which give rise to their difficulties in real life. It is certainly likely that actual association with real people in the permissive atmosphere of the consulting-room will provoke

Often called 'group analytic therapy'.

certain emotions more vividly than is possible in private session. The most frequently used intermediate technique, however, is undoubtedly interpretation. Patients are encouraged to relate the symptoms of the other members to the emotions which they see them expressing, and this probably helps them to appreciate interpretations of their own difficulties by the other patients. Another therapeutic factor is probably the way in which the knowledge that other patients experience the same disreputable feelings makes it easier for each patient to accept them in herself.

THEORETICAL EXPLANATIONS

Both practice and theory, however, differ according to the school of thought to which the psychotherapist belongs. It is interesting to see how each school tries to use the theoretical explanations evolved in private interview therapy to explain the results achieved by this new technique. Freud himself made no contribution to the technique of group psychotherapy, but devoted a short book, *Group Psychology and the Analysis of the Ego* (1921) to explaining the behaviour of crowds, armies and nations by means of his psychoanalytic model. Those of his followers who have practised group therapy, such as Slavson, usually insist that exactly the same factors are at work as in private psychoanalysis, namely 'transference relationships, catharsis, insight and/or ego-strengthening, reality-testing and sublimation'.[1] Most Freudians believe that each patient reacts to the group as she did to members of her own family in infancy, treating the therapist as she did her father or mother and the other patients as she did her brothers or sisters. S. H. Foulkes, however, who is a somewhat unorthodox Freudian, recognizes the possibility that some new therapeutic factor is introduced by this technique. He says:

> Other observers go a step further and recognize that the interaction pattern or inter-relationship between people is a new phenomenon in its own right. However, if A and B are two persons between whom this interaction takes place, it would appear to me that the presence of a third person C is required if

[1] This list is taken from *The Practice of Group Psychotherapy*, by S. R. Slavson, 1947; but 'sublimation' was added to the list in his *Analytic Group Psychotherapy*, 1950.

this inter-relationship is to be seen in perspective. This third person can compare his view of A with B's view of A; he can see A through B, or B through A, and most important, he can focus on the inter-relationship between A and B from outside, which neither A nor B can do for themselves. This model, which one might call the *model of three*, is to my mind the simplest elementary model for the understanding of inter-personal relationships. C represents that new third dimension which to my mind group observation introduces.[1]

Even here, however, Foulkes is probably saying no more than that the interaction of members of a therapeutic group allows them to see in actual operation the emotional responses which in private psychoanalysis would have to be imagined, and thus enables both therapist and patients to achieve a quicker and more thorough insight into the nature and origin of these responses. If so, Foulkes is merely explaining how group analytic therapy facilitates one of the processes in Slavson's list, namely 'insight'.

Adlerians have less difficulty in explaining the special virtue of the group. Professor Dreikurs, for example, suggests that disclosure of one's private thoughts to a group is even more beneficial than the catharsis achieved in private treatment (he points to the analogy of public confession as practised, for example, by the Buchmanites). He agrees with the Freudians that it helps 'reality-testing', but he also considers that patients are 're-educated' quicker as a result of stimulation from other members of the group. Like all Adlerians he believes, of course, in the remedial tendency of the 'community-feeling', and sees this as manifesting itself in the group in two ways. A patient feels at one with the group when she discovers that others share the feelings which she had supposed to be so abnormal; Dreikurs nick-names this 'universalization'. Patients benefit, too, from the responsibility of giving mutual help to one another. Finally, the inferiority-feeling in which Adlerians believe seems to him to be alleviated by the equalizing effect of associating patients of different status and abilities together in the same group.[2] Professor Dreikurs' list of factors at work is therefore 'catharsis, reality-testing, re-education,

---

[1] 'Group Therapy', by S. H. Foulkes, in the *British Journal of Medical Psychology*, 1950.
[2] 'Twenty Years of Group Psychotherapy', by Professor Rudolph Dreikurs and R. R. Corsini, in the *American Journal of Psychiatry*, 1954.

universalization, mutual help and equalization'. The first two agree with two of the items in the Freudian list of Slavson. The rest follow fairly naturally from the socialist view of human nature which Adler, as we saw in Chapter V, imported into psychoanalysis. Thus the Adlerians, like the Freudians, do not feel the need to recognize the operation of any really new factor in group treatment.

Analytical psychology has played very little part in the history of group psychotherapy. Jung himself regards it as a method of very limited value. He considers that while it is indispensable as a means of 'educating man as a social being', and is thus able to do what individual analysis inevitably neglects, it cannot help the individual to realize his own unique potentialities and so to become secure and self-sufficient without the support of society. He says:

> Group therapy, in my opinion, is capable only of educating the *social* side of man. In our time, when so much stress is laid on the socialization of the individual, and also because of the need for special guidance in adaptation, the formation of psychologically orientated groups certainly acquires increased importance. But owing to the notorious tendency people have of attaching themselves to others, and to -isms, instead of finding security and independence in themselves, which would be the best thing for them in the first instance, there is a danger that the individual may regard the group as his father and mother, and thereby remain as dependent, insecure and infantile as before.[1]

This rather discouraging attitude has not prevented one or two of Jung's followers, such as E. Pearl Welch in the U.S.A. and Hildebrand Teirich in Germany, from making use of this technique, and less orthodox Jungians are even readier to do so. A slightly different approach is to be found in the Jungian community founded by Mr. and Mrs. Champernowne in 1942 at Withymead in England, where patients receive individual psychotherapy on orthodox Jungian lines, with particular emphasis on the use of pictorial art, but are also intended to benefit from living, working

---

[1] From correspondence with Georg Bach and Hans Illing (1955), quoted in 'Historische Perspektive zur Gruppenpsychotherapie', by Bach and Illing, in *Zeitschrift für Psychosomatische Medizin* for January 1956 (reproduced by courtesy of Verlag für Medizinische Psychologie, Göttingen).

and carrying out other activities in the small community formed by patients and staff.[1]

I have not been able to find any clearly expressed theory about the way in which patients benefit from therapeutic communities. It is possible to believe that all the processes which Adlerians and Freudians see at work in interview groups take place, separately or in combination, in all the multitudinous contacts, however short, which the patient makes with the members of a tolerant and understanding group, and that the cumulative effect of all these contacts is large enough to be detectable. In those cases in which the patient is undergoing psychotherapy, whether in a group or in private interviews, it may be argued that these contacts provide her with better opportunities of trying out her new insight or her less repressed reactions than she would have in the more intolerant surroundings of life outside the community. Whether she is receiving psychotherapeutic treatment or not, she may benefit simply from the greater ease with which she can form friendly relationships inside such a community. It may even be suggested that man is one of those species whose needs include not merely food, drink, warmth, a mate and offspring but also a place in a group, and that someone who is deprived of this by the difficulties created by neurosis may be benefited by being placed in a group which is artificially suited to receive her.

THE FUTURE OF GROUP PSYCHOTHERAPY

Thus the beneficial properties of the group have, during the development of psychotherapy, been used in several quite distinct ways. They have been used to facilitate re-education, in 'didactic groups'; and to facilitate catharsis, in 'psychodrama'. In 'interview groups' they appear to facilitate all the processes, whatever they may be, which assist in the patient's recovery. A 'therapeutic community', on the other hand, can be regarded either as a facilitant or as itself meeting a need of the patient.

The therapeutic community, however, is not so much a definable procedure as an attitude. The scope for it appears to lie almost entirely in the handling of in-patients in mental hospitals, although it can also be used in what are called 'day hospitals', where

[1] This clearly resembles Dr. J. Bierer's device of the 'therapeutic community', mentioned earlier in this chapter.

patients who are able to live with their families but not to go to work can spend their day in remedial activities, combined with active psychotherapy. So far as active psychotherapy is concerned, the interview group seems to hold the greatest possibility of future development. It has the undoubted advantage of enabling any one psychotherapist to treat more patients at any one time, and thus reduces the cost of treatment, in terms of both money and man-power; as a result it may place psychotherapy within the reach of those who have hitherto been deprived of it either by lack of means or by shortage of practitioners. It is even possible that it is not merely a more expedient technique than the private interview but also a quicker or more effective one, if not in all types of disorder then in some. But it has one serious disadvantage, which may well prove the factor that will limit its use for some time to come. In almost all communities mental disorder, of whatever kind, is still regarded as being in some way more disreputable or contemptible than any kind of physical disorder, with the possible exception of venereal disease. When a patient is admitted to a mental hospital her family usually try to conceal her whereabouts and the nature of her illness, and even if she is able to stay at home and undergo out-patient treatment from a psychotherapist, one of her chief concerns is to conceal from her acquaintances and employers that she is doing so. Psychotherapists are therefore particularly careful not to reveal the names of their patients, and most of them take precautions to ensure that a patient does not meet another on the way to or from an interview. Obviously, however, a patient who becomes one of a group for treatment must either give up the idea of anonymity or trust to the other members of the group to preserve it. In large cities it is quite easy to form groups in which none of the patients know each other or are likely to meet each other outside the consulting-room, but the smaller the community the greater the chances of this, and even in a large city the higher the patient's position on the professional, political or social scale the more likely it is that she will be recognized. There are signs, however, that the stigma of mental illness is gradually fading, particularly in some parts of the U.S.A., and I can only hope that it will continue to do so sufficiently to allow the technique of group interview to be given a fair trial.

Recommended Reading

GROUP PSYCHOTHERAPY, by J. W. Klapman. Heinemann, 1946.

GROUP PSYCHOTHERAPY, by Rudolf Dreikurs, in the *Comptes Rendus des Séances, Premier Congres Mondial de Psychiatrie, Paris*, 1950. Hermann et Cie, 1952.

HISTORISCHE PERSPEKTIVE ZUR GRUPPENPSYCHOTHERAPIE, by G. R. Bach and H. A. Illing, in the *Zeitschrift für Psychosomatische Medizin*, 1956. (Translation to appear in the journal *Human Relations*.)

X

COMMENT AND CONCLUSION

INTERMEDIATE TECHNIQUES AND FACILITANTS

IN the preceding chapters I have tried to show how and why each school of psychotherapy has developed its particular sub-technique. They are all descended from hypnosis, which was first regarded, in the hands of Mesmer, as a curative technique in itself, but came to be recognized by the Nancy school as merely a facilitant for suggestion, a sub-technique which has survived, with and without hypnosis, to the present day. In the same way, hypnotic anamnesis, first practised by Breuer, was soon found to be merely one way of facilitating anamnesis, and in Freud's hands hypnosis was replaced as a facilitant, first by concentration and then by free association. The new intermediate techniques of interpretation and dream-interpretation, again with free association as a facilitant, were introduced by Freud a little later. Adler supplemented them with the intermediate technique of re-education, and relegated anamnesis to the status of a diagnostic questionnaire. Jung, while paying more attention to anamnesis, and making full use of interpretation and dream-interpretation, employed a more subtle form of re-education, supplemented free association with picture-painting as a facilitant for interpretation, and allowed the therapist to react less impersonally to the patient. Rogers began with a technique of diagnosis by means of psychological tests, coupled with advice to patients (or parents) about environmental questions; but gradually replaced this with a technique of interpretation that became less and less directive. Finally, some neo-Freudians in the U.S.A. use drugs or have revived hypnosis as facilitants for anamnesis. Meanwhile, as an alternative to treating patients in individual private sessions, experiments were made with grouping them together, at first as subjects for suggestion, then as classes for instruction and re-education, next as members of a body for the carrying out of communal activities, and finally as subjects for the psychotherapeutic sub-techniques which had been evolved in individual sessions.

TOPICS

The topics which have figured in psychotherapists' conversations with their patients have varied more than their intermediate techniques and facilitants. Practitioners of suggestion, with or without hypnotism, have simply selected the patients' symptoms as their topic. During the phase in which he relied chiefly on anamnesis, Freud at first chose to talk about infantile seductions, but later widened his subject to include the sexual phantasies and feelings of infancy, and then the infant's other pleasure-seeking activities; when he introduced the intermediate technique of interpretation he added the patient's defence-mechanisms and present feelings, particularly her transference-feelings towards the psychotherapist. His British followers have not added any strikingly new topics, but under the influence of Melanie Klein have paid more attention to the feelings and thoughts of early infancy, particularly oral and anal ones, whether pleasurable or aggressive. Adler preferred the topics of inferiority-feelings, the will-to-power, and the community-feeling. Partly under his influence neo-Freudians in the U.S.A. have concentrated upon inter-personal relations, and have paid less attention than their British counterparts to infantile pleasure-seeking or aggression. Jung also paid less attention to sexuality and infantile feelings, and introduced the topics of mythology, undeveloped potentialities and archetypal ways of thinking. In comparison with Freudians, Adlerians and Jungians, the followers of Rogers have no particular preference for one topic or another, unless perhaps there is a tendency to dwell on hostility to others; on the whole, the conversation is on subjects selected by the patient, which thus tend to be more obviously connected with the symptoms and difficulties of which she is conscious.

ECLECTICISM

This outline, like the rest of this book, is drawn in black and white, with sharp demarcation lines where many people would see only shades of difference. I do not think, however, that I have overdone this process. Quite apart from the fact that this book would be twice as long and half as intelligible if I had set out to define every intermediate point of view between the theories of Freud, Jung, Adler, Rogers, Coué and Moreno, it is also the case that pure exponents of the sub-techniques and theories that I have described do exist—some of them purer than their masters. On the other hand there is a growing number of psychotherapists who make an explicit point of using the intermediate techniques, facilitants and topics of more than one school. These are generally called 'eclectics'—that is, people who take their pick. So long as this designation is not used to dignify a practitioner who has not in fact had a thorough grounding in the methods of any school, the tendency is probably a healthy one. Indeed the psychotherapy of the future will probably consist of eclectic methods used in a combination of private and group interviews. The danger of eclecticism is that any success that is achieved in mild cases of neurosis by the quicker and more superficial approaches of Coué, Adler and Rogers will obscure the need, in more severe or complicated cases, for the deeper but slower methods of the Freudians and Jungians. Just as the greater hardiness and versatility of cross-bred cattle are only maintained by keeping alive the pure strains and breeding in from them occasionally, so I hope that the Freudians and Jungians will preserve their separate and belligerent stud-farms to provide bloodstock for the practical herd of the future, and will not be too tolerant of mixed marriages. Fortunately, the old bulls of the herd are seeing to this at the moment, and no doubt they will have their successors.

POPULARITY OF PSYCHOTHERAPY

A subject about which it is difficult to obtain any exact information is the extent to which psychotherapeutic methods are employed in different countries. They are of course used by many physicians and some laymen who do not belong to the professional associations of any of the main schools. At the same time, the membership of these associations in different countries should provide a rough index of the popularity of the semantic as opposed to the purely physical techniques. Fortunately the *International Journal of Psychoanalysis* provides lists of the members of almost all the various national Psychoanalytical Associations, which between them account for the vast majority of those psychotherapists who belong to any association.[1] This makes it possible to calculate the population per psychoanalyst for each country in which a Psychoanalytical Association has been formed. Even this, however, would probably be a misleading index, since an important factor which must limit the number of psychoanalysts is the number of medical practitioners[2] in any given country. The population per medical practitioner varies very greatly from one country to another, and a better index is therefore the ratio of medical practitioners to psychoanalysts. The table below shows the comparative popularity

Country[3]	Population per medical practitioner[4]		Medical practitioners[4] per psychoanalyst		Psycho-analysts[5]
		(order)		(order)	
1. Austria	646	(2)	897	(12)	12
2. Belgium	1,012	(7)	815	(11)	11
3. France	1,146	(9)	814	(10)	46
4. Germany	760	(3)	4,542	(14)	15
5. Italy	841	(5)	2,619	(13)	22
6. Netherlands	1,179	(10)	150	(3)	60
7. Sweden	1,379	(12)	187	(5)	28
8. Switzerland	999	(6)	112	(2)	44
9. Israel	431	(1)	178	(4)	22
10. Britain	1,145	(8)	303	(7)	147
11. U.S.A.	777	(4)	76	(1)	2,754
12. Argentina	1,378	(11)	277	(6)	49
13. Brazil	4,733	(14)	482	(9)	36
14. Chile	1,760	(13)	431	(8)	8

[1] Membership, for example, of associations of Individual Psychologists in the U.S.A. is estimated at about one-seventh of that of Psychoanalytical Associations.

[2] It is true that a sizeable proportion of psychoanalysts are not medically qualified, but their numbers are limited by the availability of medically qualified psychoanalysts to train and supervise them.

[3] Excluding Japan, where there is a Psychoanalytical Association whose membership had not been published at the date of going to press.

[4] Taken from 'Medical Schools and Physicians: Quantitative Aspects', by J. L. Troupin, of the *Bulletin of the World Health Organization*, 1955; his figures for medical practitioners are taken from the *United Nations Statistical Yearbook for 1954*, and include medical graduates practising any branch of medicine.

[5] Excluding honorary members of associations and those with addresses outside the country in question.

of psychoanalysis, measured by this index, in those countries for which I have been able to ascertain the membership of their Psychoanalytical Association.

It is not easy to account for the wide differences between these ratios. As the ordinal numbers in brackets show, the countries with a high ratio of physicians to population are not always those with a high ratio of psychoanalysts to physicians. It is not surprising, of course, to find very high ratios of both in Israel; ever since the Middle Ages medicine has been a favourite profession of the Jews, and the same is now true of psychoanalysis, for which they have a particular aptitude. The low ratio in Germany, Italy and Austria (the birthplace of psychoanalysis) may be connected with the totalitarian régimes of the nineteen-thirties, which were both anti-semitic and opposed to psychoanalysis. It is noticeable, however, that most of the countries with low ratios are those in which the influence of the Roman Catholic Church is strong; indeed Spain seems to have no Psychoanalytical Association at all. The Christian Churches have naturally been very suspicious of psychoanalysis, although some of the Protestant clergy—particularly Methodists—have gradually accepted it and even practised modifications of it, such as analytical psychology. The Roman Catholic Church—at least in Britain—does not officially discourage psychotherapy, although it is inevitably antagonistic to some aspects of Freudianism.[1] It is therefore possible that in countries with a large Catholic population the small membership of Psychoanalytical Associations does not accurately reflect the popularity of psychotherapeutic techniques of all kinds, and is counter-balanced by the popularity of non-Freudian methods. I am inclined to think, however, that this is only part of the explanation, and that a predominantly Catholic population is to some extent less favourable to psychotherapy, either because resort to it is considered inconsistent with their faith or because the incidence of neurosis and allied disorders is lower than in non-Catholic populations. This is, however, a pure conjecture, which may have overlooked other important factors.

[1] See, for example, the Catholic Truth Society's pamphlet *Psychoanalysis and Other Aspects of Psychology*, by C. L. C. Burns, M.R.C.S., D.P.M., 1955.

EFFICACY

Another question which is bound to be asked by every reader is 'Which sub-technique is the most effective?' There are one or two places where I have mentioned the shortcomings of some procedure (such as suggestion) in order to explain why psychotherapists looked for some way of improving on it. But with these few exceptions I have deliberately reserved the question of the comparative efficacy of Freudian, Adlerian, Jungian or Rogerian treatment for this final chapter, and even here I have nothing very conclusive to say.

In the first place, doubt has been cast on the efficacy of any of these forms of psychotherapy. Psychoanalysis was of course attacked from the start on religious, moral, philosophical and occasionally scientific grounds.[1] More recently, its effectiveness has been denied by writers with a personal stake in some other sub-technique,[2] but without any very conclusive arguments. In 1952, however, H. J. Eysenck, of the London University Institute of Psychiatry, published in a short article[3] an argument based on a much more serious and impartial study. After collating the results of treatment in 7,293 cases as reported in 5 articles by psychoanalysts and 19 articles by 'eclectic' psychotherapists, he found that the average proportion of those classified as 'cured', 'much improved' or 'improved' was two-thirds of the patients treated. He compared this with the recovery rate in two groups of neurotics which were assumed to have had no treatment. Among the cases of severe neurosis admitted to New York State Hospitals the proportion discharged annually as 'recovered or improved' between 1925 and 1934 was just over two-thirds. The other group consisted of five hundred neurotics whose claims for disability were taken from the files of the Equitable Life Assurance Society in the U.S.A.; the only treatment they received consisted of sedatives, tonics, suggestion or reassurance from their own physi-

---

[1] See, for example, *A Critical Examination of Psychoanalysis*, by A. Wohlgemuth, 1921, and *The Successful Error*, by R. Allers, 1941.

[2] See, for example, *The Case Against Psychoanalysis*, by A. Salter, 1952, whose own suggestive sub-technique is described in Chapter VIII.

[3] In the *Journal of Consulting Psychology*, 1952. A popular exposition of his statistics will be found in Chapter 10 of his book *The Uses and Abuses of Psychology*, 1953. His article was criticized by Lester Luborsky of the Menninger Foundation, in the U.S.A., in the *British Journal of Psychology*, 1954, which also contains a rejoinder by Eysenck.

cians. A follow-up over periods of five to ten years showed that after one year 45 per cent, after two years 72 per cent and after five years 90 per cent had returned to work, complained of no further or very slight difficulties and had made successful social adjustments. Eysenck summed up his paper thus:

> The figures fail to support the hypothesis that psychotherapy facilitates recovery from neurotic disorder. In view of the many difficulties attending such actuarial comparisons, no further conclusions could be derived from the data, whose shortcomings high-light the necessity of properly planned and executed experimental studies into this important field.

This paper has been mistaken for an attempt to prove that the treatment of neurosis by psychotherapy does not produce a higher recovery-rate than would occur naturally and without intervention. In fact, as Eysenck was the first to admit, it merely shows that the only statistics he could find did not suggest a higher recovery rate as a result of psychotherapy; and he himself emphasized the imperfections of his 'control groups' of untreated neurotics. Among the defects of his statistics are the following:

(a) neither of the control groups were completely untreated;

(b) the statistics for the controls may have been significantly affected by the neurotics' motives for presenting themselves as 'ill' or 'improved'. For example, a hospitalized neurotic might decide that he would rather be neurotic outside than inside an institution and might therefore say he was 'better'. An insurance-claimant, too, might make the most of a slight disability if he saw a profit in it, but become tired, ashamed or frightened of keeping it up for too long;

(c) the physicians in charge of the controls may also have had motives for deciding when they were 'improved'. All public hospitals for mental and physical disorders have to meet such heavy demands for beds that they have strong incentives to discharge patients as soon as they safely can;

(d) on the other hand there is the probability that patients who seek out-patient psychotherapy instead of being admitted to hospital are not so severely ill, and therefore have less room for improvement. This might also account for the high recovery rate among the insurance-claimants, although this is less likely;

(e) in collating the results reported by psychotherapists, Eysenck has counted patients who died as being in the same category as those who showed 'no improvement'; he allowed for those who broke off treatment in referring to the results of psychoanalysis, but not in the case of other types of psychotherapy. His papers do not show how serious or trivial the effect of this may have been;

(f) over 60 per cent of the patients treated by psychoanalysis belonged to a single very old sample from the Berlin Psychoanalytic Institute, and were treated in the nineteen-twenties, in many cases by trainee analysts taking their first cases;

(g) neurosis may, like some other mental disorders, be a cyclic condition, with remissions and relapses even when it is not treated; it is not clear to what extent this possibility was guarded against in the case either of the controls or of the treated patients;

(h) it would not be surprising if a high proportion of those who seek psychotherapeutic treatment were drawn from the group who do not improve spontaneously.[1]

I am not arguing, however, that Eysenck's paper is unimportant. It does in fact suggest the possibility that 'roughly two-thirds of a group of neurotic patients will recover or improve to a marked extent within about two years of the onset of their illness, whether they are treated by means of psychotherapy or not'.[2] So far as I know this still requires proper statistical confirmation, which must exclude the possibility that neurosis is a cyclic condition. This could only be done by a follow-up of a large number of cases over several years, with objective tests for severity and improvement of the various kinds of neurosis. But if it did confirm Eysenck's hypothesis, it would mean that psychotherapists would either have to show a better score than 66 per cent (or whatever percentage the investigation yielded), or prove that they were drawing their patients mainly from those who do not spontaneously improve. Even so, there would still be a risk of oversimplifying the issue.

[1] I owe some of these points—(d), (e) and (f)—to Lester Luborsky (loc. cit.) although he did not put them in this precise form. Point (a) is, I rather think, admitted by Eysenck himself. So far as I know he has not commented on points (e) or (f) although he replied to Luborsky in the same issue.

[2] Eysenck claims that his statistics 'show' this, but in view of the points I have listed I think this is going too far.

It might not be sufficiently precise to think in terms of a patient being treated for a disorder by a psychotherapist. There are many kinds of patients, disorders, psychotherapists and, as the previous chapters have shown, sub-techniques. Let us consider some of these differences.

THE PATIENT

Patients vary in innumerable respects, and there is every probability that some of these affect their chances of cure by semantic sub-techniques, to say nothing of spontaneous recovery. The factors most likely to be relevant are

Age: there is probably an age, varying from person to person, after which her response to psychotherapy becomes progressively slower and and probably also less marked.

Intelligence: a certain level of intelligence is of course required to make semantic methods possible at all. The language and topics of some schools (such as the Jungian) make more demands on the intelligence and education of the patient than do others (such as the Rogerian): but this does not necessarily mean that their results are better.

Sex: it is possible that one sex may respond better to psychotherapy than the other. A recent survey by Dr. Rosenbaum and others in Cincinnati, U.S.A.,[1] found that more men than women broke off treatment before completion, but found no other sex-difference in the proportions of 'improved' patients.

Personality: some types of personality may respond quicker or better to psychotherapy than others. There is still very little agreement among psychologists about the definition of basic traits, but most are agreed that 'suggestibility', for example, is one. Eysenck found a high correlation between a particular kind of suggestibility and 'neuroticism' in 1,000 male servicemen suffering from neurosis,[2] but because he did not administer psychotherapy there is no indication whether the more suggestible patients would have

---

[1] Dr. M. Rosenbaum *et alii*, 'Evaluation of Results of Psychotherapy' in the journal *Psychosomatic Medicine*, 1956, which again reported just over two-thirds of its patients as 'improved'.

[2] See *Dimensions of Personality*, 1947.

responded to it quicker or better. Rosenbaum's survey found that the less 'religious' patients tended to improve more; but most psychologists would prefer to look for some more precisely definable trait than this.

Circumstances: although psychotherapy aims at altering the patient and not her environment, the latter must often be relevant. An alcoholic may have an unsatisfactory spouse, a frustrating job or a disability that prevents her from living a normal life; and these will make it harder for her to respond to treatment of her own defects of character.

THE DISORDER

As we saw in Chapter II, psychotherapy began by being a remedial technique for certain physical symptoms, such as hysterical paralyses, but was extended by Freud to treat anxiety states, obsessions and perversions. Some examples of the sort of disorder which are quite often (though not of course always) treated by psychotherapy nowadays are

Physical symptoms:
    hysterical paralyses, tics and convulsions
    asthma
    dyspareunia, frigidity, impotence, ejaculatio praecox
    anorexia nervosa
    enuresis
    psychogenic vomiting
    psychogenic headache
Anxiety states:
    claustrophobia and agoraphobia
    hypochondria
    insomnia
Behaviour disorders:
    alcoholism and other addictions
    homosexuality and other perversions
    kleptomania and other compulsive behaviour
    delinquency (in children and adolescents)
Psychoses
    schizophrenia
    depressive states

Not all psychotherapeutic schools would attempt of course to treat all these disorders. Most psychotherapists, for example, would be cautious about the prospects of cure in cases of homosexuality, psychosis or delinquency, particularly in older patients. Jung would point out that 'about a third of my cases are not suffering from any clinically definable neurosis, but from the senselessness and aimlessness of their lives' (see Chapter VI). It seems to me highly probable that in some of the disorders I have listed a large-scale survey would find that the psychotherapist's score was very much higher than the spontaneous improvement-rate, while in others it was no higher (and might conceivably be lower). I am not of course arguing from this that psychotherapists should take on only those patients or disorders which are suspected to have good prospects of improvement, simply in order to score as high as possible. This might mean withholding from a would-be patient his only remaining hope of salvation. But in cases where the available evidence suggests that the prospects under psychotherapy are not bright, and that other techniques, such as those of physical medicine, have beneficial effects, the psychotherapist owes it to his patient and the reputation of his own profession to consider whether these other techniques should not first be tried.

THE PSYCHOTHERAPIST

Psychotherapists vary in age and intelligence, just as patients do, although they probably tend less to extremes in these respects. They also vary in training and experience. On the whole, however, their personal traits are probably of most importance in affecting the success of treatment. Just as some people are 'natural' or 'born' leaders, orators or practitioners of other semantic techniques, so there seem to be people who have, irrespective of their training and their theories, an unlearned ability to treat people by one psychotherapeutic sub-technique or another. Sometimes they are, like stage hypnotists, good at 'suggestion', and can inspire confidence and impart reassurance, particularly when invested with the authority of a consulting-room. Others are good at 'drawing people out', and inducing them to talk freely about themselves. Others are good at explaining people to themselves in clear and convincing terms. A fourth group, rarer than any of the others, combine these abilities. A fifth group possess none of them, but are occasionally impelled to train as psychotherapists; these have to rely either on the learning of rules or on imitation of their instructors. Some of these groups—for example, the last—will probably score a smaller proportion of successes than the others. The very high demand, however, for treatment of the sort of disorders I have listed means that there are too few psychotherapists to meet it, and so long as this is so there will be insufficient competition to ensure the survival of the good ones. In this situation the only factor that can operate to eliminate bad ones is a high standard of selection in the training institutions. There is no doubt that the reputable institutions do exercise their powers of selection, but our notions of what makes a good or a bad psychotherapist are still crude and unscientific. Very little attention, for example, has been paid to the question of the sex of the psychotherapist and the patient. In view of the Freudians' theories about the Oedipus complex and the transference, they might be expected to have considered very seriously whether the patient and the psychotherapist should be of opposite sexes, if not in all disorders, then in some. Since a person's sex is one of the few characteristics about which there is no controversy among psychologists or psychotherapists, this should be a point on which a statistical survey could throw light: but so far as I know none has been carried out.

THE SUB-TECHNIQUE

Any survey, therefore, which set out to compare the efficacy of the different sub-techniques would have to find some way of eliminating the uncertainties arising from the varieties of patient, of disorder and of psychotherapist, while at the same time leaving a large enough sample to support its conclusions. For example, the total number of patients in the age-group 21–25 under any kind of psychotherapeutic treatment for claustrophobia at any one time in Britain is small, and may be too small to allow it to be subdivided for statistical comparison into those being treated by Freudians, those being treated by Adlerians and so on; and even this subdivision would take no account of some of the variables I have mentioned. What is more, the present tendency towards eclecticism, although probably healthy from other points of view, could reach a stage at which distinctions between the methods of different psychotherapists could not be drawn with sufficient precision for a comparison of this kind.

My own guess, which is based on nothing more than a study of the literature and conversations with psychotherapists of different schools and some of their patients, is that if it were ever possible to carry out a proper survey it would show that the approaches of different schools were suited to different types of patient and disorder. Jung himself, for example, said 'fully two-thirds of my patients are in the second half of life' and it is possible that his sub-technique with its topics and explanatory model, is better suited than others to deal with the difficulties of middle and old age. The topics and intermediate techniques of psychoanalysis may be better suited to the first half of life, when sexuality is one of the most important forces to be taken into account. There may be certain disorders, for example, in the malleable period of adolescence, which will respond satisfactorily to the shorter and less deep sub-techniques, such as those of Rogers or Adler. Some disorders, whatever the patient's age, may respond better or quicker to group therapy than to individual sessions. These are, however, nothing more than hypotheses, based on no statistical evidence, and put forward merely as examples of what might some day be established.

In the meantime, what determines the type of psychotherapist who treats a particular patient? In private practice, it is very often the choice of the patient herself. She may have heard of the success of a particular practitioner with some other case, and although her own disorder or circumstances may be different she may decide to consult him. Or she may have read about the topics emphasized by the different schools, and may feel that one sounds more congenial or less embarrassing than another. Even if she consults her family doctor (and most psychotherapists prefer that he should know they are treating her) his choice cannot often be based on practical experience, although it is likely to be sounder than her own. A better method is a long diagnostic interview with a psychotherapist who has an impartial acquaintance not only with the different sub-techniques (physical as well as semantic) but also with the local practitioners of them, and who assigns the patient to one of these practitioners. Some clinics in Britain and the U.S.A. are able to provide a service of this kind, and it is a tendency which may well become more widespread.

THE NATURE OF PSYCHOTHERAPEUTIC CURE

Another question which may trouble someone who has read the rest of this book is 'How do these sub-techniques cure or alleviate the disorder?' Here again what I have to say is very tentative.

There are first of all the technical explanations of the psychotherapists themselves. We have seen how the suggestive school explained their results, first in terms of the ideo-motor model and more recently in terms of 'conditioning'. Freud's original cathartic explanation of the beneficial effects of anamnesis was also based on the ideo-motor model, and visualized traumatic memories as being removed from the unconscious like a foreign body swallowed by a child. When he introduced the intermediate techniques of interpretation, he began to assign a positive function to the conscious ego, and ego-analysis and transference-analysis are conceived of by Freudians as in some way altering it; the patient's ego is 'strengthened', she achieves 'insight' into what she wants and feels, and at the same time is more realistic about what she can actually have and do. Adler, who had very little use for the model of the unconscious, saw the process as one of arguing with the patient and re-educating her into a less anti-social way of living. Rogers sees it as mainly the achievement of 'insight', although he also allows a part to the 'release of expression', which seems to be his description of the Freudian catharsis. Jung regards his method as developing the patient's undeveloped potentialities and enabling her to recognize and come to terms with the ways in which her thoughts and behaviour are governed by her ancestral history. Finally, we have seen that psychotherapists are now realizing that their explanations must also explain the beneficial effects of group methods.

Psychologists have also offered explanations of the effects of psychotherapy in terms of their scientific models. The nineteenth-century ideo-motor model might be regarded as having been a scientific one before it was taken over by the early psychotherapists of France. More modern psychological explanations, as we saw in Chapter VIII, are in terms either of learning theory, or occasionally, of 'conditioned reflexes'.

Some explanations give a greater intellectual satisfaction than others. It is particularly satisfying when someone describes a mysterious process in terms of some phenomenon with which we are familiar; the pleasure is probably the same as children get from hearing a story that they have heard before. If psychotherapeutic cures can be described in terms of something which we come across every day—for example, as a kind of learning or relearning—we are pleasantly relieved that we do not have to add a new and unfamiliar kind of phenomenon to our list. This satisfaction is not necessarily irrelevant from either the scientific or the technical point of view. It is unscientific to create a new class of phenomena when an existing one will serve; and it is technically useful to have an explanation which patients will understand and accept. But from this point the scientist's and the technician's needs begin to diverge. The former wants an explanation that will not only link psychotherapeutic cures to other phenomena of human behaviour, but will also cover all the facts that can be observed about those cures. It must, for example, make plausible

- (i) the effects of suggestion, anamnesis and interpretation;
- (ii) the effects of group treatment;
- (iii) the need for a certain level of intelligence in the patient;
- (iv) the phenomena of transference;
- (v) the importance of the patient's age;
- (vi) the importance of certain topics, and the irrelevance of others;
- (vii) the variation in length of treatment with different patients, disorders and sub-techniques;
- (viii) the possibility of spontaneous improvement.

In contrast, the technician requires an explanation that will tell him what to do in the particular case with which he is dealing; in other words, that will tell him what to say and how to say it; and that will tell him this quickly, so that he does not have to pause for calculation before replying to his patient. To get an explanation of this sort he may have to sacrifice some of the scope and precision of the scientific explanation, and may have to be content with one that suits the sort of case he is dealing with but would not suit another. Again, the sort of explanation that would be of help in applying the intermediate technique of anamnesis might be of less use in the intermediate technique of re-education. So that unless a psychotherapist confines himself to one type of patient and one intermediate technique, it is unlikely that his explanations will be of the kind to fit together into a tidy and comprehensive system like that of the scientist; and this is, I think, exactly what we find. The explanatory models of the Freudian, Adlerian or Jungian are less consistent than those of the laboratory psychologists, and explain only limited sectors of human behaviour. But this does not mean that they are merely inferior kinds of psychological explanation: they were evolved in the consulting-room for the purpose of treating patients, a practical task for which the models of the laboratory are of little value.

I should like, nevertheless, to offer a personal comment which is neither a psychotherapeutic nor a scientific explanation, but which may make the phenomena of psychotherapy seem less mysterious. Long before Freud was born it was realized that the child is father of the man, and could be taught both ways of behaving and facts much more easily than an adult. Parents, nurses and schoolteachers have never hesitated to take the credit for inculcating any good qualities which he might later exhibit. If his defects were more obvious than his virtues they regarded them as inborn, and blamed themselves for not eradicating them more thoroughly. Freud's technique for treating the physical symptoms of hysteria led him to realize that defects of personality as well as virtues could be the result of upbringing. Gradually he and his followers[1] came to appreciate how much the success of their methods depended on the personal relationship between psychotherapist and patient—that is, on the transference. As naturalists know, the young of most warm-blooded animals, however well-cared-for, seem to require the presence of a parent for the proper development of their normal patterns of behaviour, and studies of children who have been separated—for example, by war—from their mothers suggest that, however well they are cared for materially, they quickly deteriorate psychologically and even physically, unless a foster-parent is almost immediately found to take her place.[2] Naturalists such as Lorentz have pointed out that in some animals—such as wild or domesticated dogs—this need and capacity for attachment to a quasi-parental object persists into adult-

---

[1] That is, Freudians and neo-Freudians. Jungians are equally alive to the importance of the transference. Adlerians and Rogerians are not.

[2] See, for example, *Child Care and the Growth of Love*, by Dr. J. Bowlby, 1950.

hood. Long before this, however, Freud noticed the similarity between the transference and the child's relationship to his parents. It seems to me very probable that the transference, if properly handled by the psychotherapist, in some way rectifies the defects of the patient's original relationship with one or both of her parents.[1] We have seen in earlier chapters how much importance the schools of psychotherapy have attached to the different intermediate techniques—anamnesis, interpretation, re-education—and how the transference was regarded first as a nuisance (by Breuer, the young Freud and to some extent Adler), and later as a facilitant for the intermediate techniques which really effected the cure. We have seen, too, how much importance each school—with the exception of Rogers'—attaches to the discussion of particular topics; and how modern psychoanalysis makes the transference an essential topic. It seems to me extremely probable that the transference is more than a facilitant and more than a topic, and that the establishment and proper handling of this relationship is an intermediate technique in itself. It is even possible that what have been regarded by psychotherapists as intermediate techniques which are facilitated by the transference are in some cases really facilitants for the transference; the anamnesis, for example, of childhood experiences may not be a catharsis so much as a means of intensifying the similarity between the transference and the parent-child relationship. It may of course be argued that a psychotherapist who does not believe in the importance of the transference may nevertheless achieve results. But the example of Mesmer shows that it is possible to achieve results with a quite mistaken theory about the way in which one is doing it.

*   *   *   *   *

This book is the history of a technique, and I have said nothing about the influence of psychotherapeutic theories upon our ways of thought on other subjects, such as religion, morals, law, art and literature. Freud himself warned his followers against making psychoanalysis the basis for a philosophy of life: but through no fault of his it seems to have appeared at the right time to meet a need. The discoveries of science had extended the domain of

---

[1] I owe this suggestion to 'The Therapeutic Factor in Psychotherapy', by H. Guntrip, B.D., Ph.D., in the *British Journal of Medical Psychology*, 1953.

realism and materialism over all natural phenomena with the exception of human behaviour. In this field the models of the neurologists and laboratory psychologists had offered hopes of an eventual conquest but had not yet fulfilled them. Freud's technical discoveries were explained by him in terms of a model which was copied from the feelings and thoughts familiar to everyday introspection. Like the discovery of perspective by the early Italian painters it seemed to turn a world of two dimensions into one of three dimensions, and to explain what had previously seemed meaningless. In spite of the limitations I have emphasized, his model was seized by the realists and materialists and carried like a banner into all the battlefields of humanism. Freud himself, in spite of his own warning, could not resist the temptation to apply his theories to the dissection of literature, art and religious belief, and he was soon imitated and outdone by his enthusiastic followers. In comparison, the theories of Adler, Jung and Fromm had a much smaller effect; no doubt the reason was partly that they had so much in common with Freud and partly that what they added was really dictated, as we have seen, by political, mythological or sociological interests, and had less chance of being so widely applied. However this may be, the total number of psychotherapists has always been small, and the patients they can treat can never be more than a negligible fraction of mankind. The importance, therefore, of the indirect influence of psychotherapy upon priests, clergymen, lawyers, teachers, writers, critics and philosophers must have been very largely due to their own vaguely felt need for a new approach to their problems. The psychotherapists were eager to accept any invitations, and like other welcome guests sometimes overstayed their welcome; but they made a lasting impression on their hosts.

All that, however, is another story. Whatever the implications of psychotherapy for other fields of knowledge, it is itself nothing more than the semantic group of remedial techniques for treating psychogenic disorders. Its future will obviously depend on two things. One is the extent to which non-semantic techniques, using drugs or surgery or other devices, succeed in providing quick, effective and lasting remedies for one kind of neurosis or another, without detriment to the patient. My own belief is that we shall see advances in this direction, but that they will never reach a point at which non-semantic techniques are sensitive enough to alleviate all the more subtle maladjustments of the delicate human machine. Thus there will always be scope for psychotherapy. It may be limited to fewer disorders than those it is forced, for want of anything better, to attempt to treat today. But this should enable it not only to develop the most effective techniques for treating these remaining disorders, but also to make itself available to many sufferers from them who cannot, through sheer numbers, be treated properly today.

APPENDIX A

Child Psychotherapy

THE main part of this short book has been confined to the development of techniques (and their intermediate techniques) for the psychotherapy of adults, and I have referred to the treatment of children only where this has clearly had an effect upon those techniques: examples have been the influence of Mrs. Klein's experience with children upon her method of treating adults, or the way in which the interview group technique grew out of the treatment of children and adolescents by Adler and Slavson. This brief appendix merely sketches the development of modern child therapy, and indicates the important respects in which its methods differ from those used with adults.

For a long time the differences between the minds of children and adults were not appreciated. In the eighteenth century in Britain boys of twelve were sent to Universities or hung for theft. Like adults, children became the subject of psychological studies some time before any psychotherapeutic technique was devised for treating their disorders. In the eighteen-sixties Sir Francis Galton, in his anthropometric laboratory at University College, London, made 'measurements' of children at the request of parents and teachers 'to learn their powers' or to 'obtain timely warnings of remediable faults in their development'; but it was left to the parent or teacher to deal in their own ways with such faults, and the methods they employed were no doubt didactic or disciplinary. It was not neurosis in children, but delinquency, that brought home to their elders the need for some special technique of dealing with psychogenic symptoms. The technique first used was not unnaturally that of hypnotic suggestion. In 1889 Dr. Berillon submitted to the International Congress of Hypnotism in Paris a paper on 'The Value of Hypnotism in the Treatment of Vicious and Degenerate Children'. He seems to have used it as an auxiliary in the moral re-education of lying, cruel, idle and timid children, and to have employed it as his main instrument in the cure of incontinence of urine or faeces, night terrors and masturbation.

The hypnotic and suggestive methods of Liébeault and Coué were used with children as with adults, and as recently as 1949, Mr. J. G. Ambrose reported the use of hypnotism in dealing with children at the Prince of Wales Hospital in Tottenham, London. Cases which he described included bed-wetting, faecal incontinence, sleep-walking and night terrors. He added, however, that 'hypnosis was used simply as a reinforcement for psychotherapy aimed principally at the parents of the children treated'.[1] Like the nineteenth-century French practitioners, he finds that children are particularly easy to hypnotize, does not seem to think that it does them any harm, and does not use any technique which is not common in the hypnotic treatment of adults.

One of the first clinics set up to treat rather than study children must have been the Chicago Juvenile Psychopathic Clinic, which opened in 1909; once more it was the delinquent child who was the subject. It was followed in 1915 by the famous Judge Baker Clinic in Boston. The methods employed were still those of training and education, and it was some considerable time before the influence of psychoanalysis began to make itself felt in this field.

Although Freud's technique was very largely one for reducing the ill-effects of childhood upon the adult, and although he himself was an acute observer of children's behaviour, he did not treat children. It is true that one of his classic case-histories is that of the cure of a phobia in a five-year-old boy called Hans; but Freud himself saw the boy only once, and the treatment in fact took the form of cross-questioning by the boy's father, who reported the results to Freud. He used the case to support several of his conclusions about the formation of neurosis in childhood, but actually dismissed the possibility of psychoanalysing children in his opening paragraph:

> No-one else [but the father], in my opinion, could possibly have prevailed on the child to make such avowals. The special knowledge by means of which the father was able to interpret the remarks made by his five-year-old son was indispensable, and without it the technical difficulties in the way of conducting

---

[1] 'Hypnosis: its Value in Child Guidance', by J. G. Ambrose, L.M.S.S.A, in the *British Journal of Medical Hypnotism*, 1949, to whom I am indebted for the account of Berillon's paper.

psychoanalysis with so young a child would have been insuperable. It was only because the authority of a father and a physician were united in a single person, and because in him both affectionate care and scientific interest were combined, that it was possible *in this one instance* to apply the method to a use to which it would not otherwise have lent itself.[1]

The first person to have treated children by psychoanalytic methods seems to have been Frau Dr. Hermine von Hug-Hellmuth, a member of the Vienna Psychoanalytic Society. She did not treat children under the age of six, and this was probably deliberate, since Freudians believed that it was at this age that children began to repress their infantile sexual feelings and interests, and entered the 'latency period'. Certainly there seems to have been a feeling that there were dangers as well as difficulties in psychoanalysing children before that age. Dr. Hug-Hellmuth apparently employed the intermediate techniques normally used in the psychoanalytic treatment of adults, but occasionally induced the child to draw or play with toys.

It was probably Mrs. Melanie Klein, however, who made the first important technical innovation to suit the method to children. After studying psychoanalysis under Ferenczi in Budapest and being psychoanalysed, she began to treat children in Berlin in 1919, where she was influenced by Karl Abraham.[2] She found that children are unable to co-operate as well as adults in the intermediate technique of free association, so that one of the main methods of revealing unconscious feelings to the patient and analyst is virtually closed. This led her to modify the usual technique in at least two important respects. She provided her child-patients with toys, and used the ways in which they played with them as data for her inferences about the unconscious forces at work in them. The child is allowed, for example, to play with toys which can represent its father, mother or siblings, and with water and mud which obviously resemble urine and faeces, and its manner of playing with these is regarded as a clear indication of its attitude to the objects which these represent. Mrs. Klein also found that Ferenczi's tendency to force interpretations on his patients was

[1] 'Analysis of a Phobia in a Five-year-old Boy', 1909 (*Collected Papers*, Vol. III). The italics are Freud's. (Reproduced by courtesy of the Hogarth Press.)
[2] I owe this information to a personal communication from her.

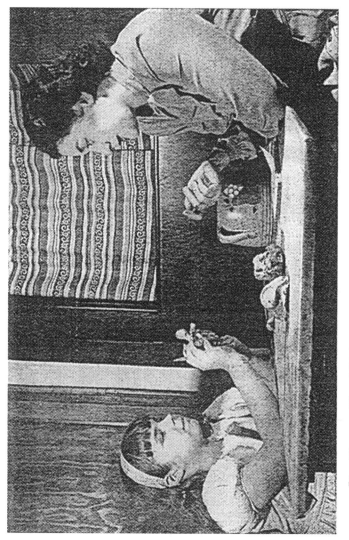

Play Therapy. The child (a volunteer and not a genuine patient) makes a clay man while the psychotherapist listens and watches her behaviour towards it.

[to face page 170

helpful with patients who were too young either to put their feelings into words or to be convinced of them by subtler methods. These innovations greatly lessened the obvious practical difficulties of treating children under six years of age, and Mrs. Klein does not seem to have had any doubts about the wisdom of doing so; her recorded cases include infants of less than three years.

Mrs. Klein's technique of 'play therapy', as it is now called, has been adopted with various modifications by the followers of Freud, Adler, Jung and Rogers, in the child guidance clinics which have been set up in all the large cities of Western Europe and the U.S.A. Their interpretations vary, of course, according to their different theories, and there are one or two technical differences. For example, in the Hampstead Clinic in London, run by Freud's youngest daughter, Anna Freud, children play with toys but not with water and mud, on the grounds that it affords too direct a gratification and therefore hinders the therapeutic process—a view which obviously resembles the Freudian doctrine that treatment should be carried out in a 'state of abstinence' (see Chapter VII). There are a number of disagreements, largely theoretical, over the part played by transference in the treatment of children; almost all schools recognize that a child develops a strong attachment to its therapist (and also a certain amount of antagonism), and make use of this to assist treatment, but there is also a school of thought which attaches little importance to the transference and sees no harm in frequent changes of therapist. Dr. Margaret Lowenfeld seems to have been first to see that the child's play is not only valuable as material for interpretation but also a process which has a therapeutic effect of its own; a belief which is supported by the beneficial effect of 'occupational therapy' on adults, although this may not be an exact analogy.

Slavson's New York clinic was probably the first, in the early nineteen-thirties, to make any large-scale use of group methods in the treatment of children, and I have described in Chapter IX how it played an important part in the development of this technique for adults.[1] Moreno's technique of psychodrama, which is also described in Chapter IX, was developed with children as one

[1] Adler's so-called group treatment of children in the nineteen-twenties, which I have described in Chapter IX, was more like a public individual session with each child in front of parents and teachers.

of the main types of patient, although he justified this by the mistaken argument that children, unlike adults, could not form a transference to a psychotherapist and so required a special technique.

Although Adler's contribution to the history of child psychotherapy cannot go unmentioned, it has probably done less than that of Mrs. Klein to shape modern technique. It was of course as a result of his efforts and those of his followers that child guidance clinics were established, first in Vienna and gradually in other cities of Europe, the U.S.A. and finally Britain. His methods, however, which involved, as we have seen, a good deal of re-education and a public interview with the child in front of its parents, are now less popular than they were. It is, for example, generally recognized that children will talk more freely about their difficulties if their parents are not present. On the other hand, Adler was probably the first to recognize the need to deal with parents, whose behaviour or attitude towards the child may be primarily responsible for its symptoms.[1] In this he was followed by the early counsellors, who, as we have seen, attached more importance to the modification of the environment than to the treatment of the patient. Most modern child guidance clinics, while treating the child, also try at least to advise the mother about her handling of it, and some give interviews to parents at which they are more or less under treatment themselves, whether they appreciate it or not. It was also Adler who recognized the effect upon a child's personality of its place in the order of children in its family: firstborn, last-born and only children each have their own peculiar difficulties.

These developments do not of course mean that the psychotherapeutic methods used with adults have been abandoned for children. All schools would agree that there comes a point at which the child's capacity to express feelings verbally has matured sufficiently to make adult psychoanalytic methods more effective than play techniques; with some children this stage is reached earlier than with others.

Child psychotherapy is a field in which the merits of the non-medical therapist are undisputed, even in the U.S.A. Most child psychotherapists are women, who not only derive particular satis-

---

[1] It is occasionally necessary to explain tactfully to parents that it is not their child's behaviour but their own attitude to it that is abnormal. Too many people still judge children by adult standards.

faction from working with children but also seem to secure a quicker response from young children than men can. Many of these women have a University degree or diploma in psychology, but work under the general supervision of a psychotherapist with a medical qualification.

Recommended Reading

AN INTRODUCTION TO CHILD GUIDANCE, by W. M. Burbury, E. M. Balint and B. J. Yapp. Macmillan, 1950.

APPENDIX B

Psychosomatic Medicine

AN important by-product of psychotherapy is psychosomatic medicine. Although psychotherapy began as a technique for treating the apparently physical or 'somatic' symptoms of hysteria, it soon achieved recognition as a method of treating mental or 'psychic' symptoms such as phobias. Many nineteenth-century physicians, however, who had never heard of Freud were convinced that a large number of apparently somatic disorders arose from or were aggravated by psychic causes, and the term 'psychosomatic' was used to describe these hybrids.[1] This classification was based of course on Descartes' separation of mind and body as two kinds of substance, the former being non-spatial ('unextended') and invisible, the latter being spatial, tangible and visible; this had been adopted as the official view of Protestantism, under the impression that it was the only metaphysical view which was reconcilable with the Christian notion of an immortal soul. But the rapid development of science—and particularly physiology —during the nineteenth century was inevitably accompanied by a materialistic attitude towards the mind-body relationship, and most physicians and psychiatrists came to regard psychic phenomena as mere accompaniments ('epiphenomena', as T. H. Huxley called them) to the working of a purely physical machine; so that the causes of even psychic disorders were sought for among the nervous, endocrine, digestive and other systems of the body.

The methods of Bernheim, Freud and Coué, however, which apparently involved no interference with the bodily machine, seemed to show that the mind was more than a mere accompaniment to the workings of that machine, and that faulty functioning of the machine, such as hysterical paralysis or vomiting, could be rectified by influencing the mind. Hitherto the theorists who

[1] See 'Psychosomatic Medicine in the Nineteenth Century', by E. Stainbrook, in the journal *Psychosomatic Medicine* for May/June, 1952.

believed in the psychic origin of some somatic disorders had been unable to make any practical use of their theory through lack of any idea of how to treat the mind instead of the body; but the two techniques of suggestion and psychoanalysis seemed to put theory into practice.

Coué, as we have seen in Chapter VIII, used his method to treat a very wide range of somatic disorders, although the results were not always very lasting.

Although Freud himself—and many of his patients—suffered from disorders which would now be called psychosomatic, he was more interested in the relief of psychic disorder, and the use of psychoanalysis as a means of treating somatic disorder was first attempted by Georg Groddeck (1866–1934), a German physician, who came into contact with Freud during the first world war. He had already come to the conclusion that many of the physical symptoms which distressed his patients took their precise form because of the way in which they symbolized unconscious desires; he believed, for example, that the vomiting of early pregnancy was due to a desire to eject the child. Until he met Freud, however, he had no technical means, beyond suggestion and some interpretation, of treating such symptoms, and it was not until then that he began to use psychoanalytic methods. Not having been trained or analysed by a Freudian, he was regarded as unorthodox in his methods, but succeeded in stimulating physicians and psychotherapists in both Germany and Britain to a similar approach towards many somatic disorders.[1]

The result has been, broadly speaking, that the suggestive method has tended to become less popular, as a means of treating somatic disorder; it is chiefly used as an accompaniment to the administration of sedatives or placebos by physicians with no pretensions to psychotherapeutic training who are treating mild symptoms with no discoverable somatic cause. For the more persistent and troublesome symptoms of this kind non-suggestive psychotherapeutic treatment has become increasingly popular. Where it is successful, its effect seems to be to replace the physical

[1] Groddeck had of course an influence on Freud, for it was from him that Freud derived the concept of the 'id' (see Chapter III). It is said that Groddeck himself owed this concept to Nietzsche, but it is interesting to see (from the translator's preface to Groddeck's *The World of Man* (tr. M. Collins, 1934)) that Nietzsche is said to have been influenced by the writings of Groddeck's father.

symptoms by conscious emotional conflict, which usually yields in its turn to further psychotherapeutic treatment.

The scientific study of somatic disorders from the psychological point of view has become correspondingly fashionable. Statistical studies of the temperaments and behaviour of sufferers from various kinds of disorder[1] have shown that particular types of personality have a tendency to be associated with a particular kind of somatic disorder. For example, four separate investigations arrived at the conclusion that a very high proportion of sufferers from ulcerative colitis shared the following traits—'emotional immaturity, fearfulness and attacks that were precipitated when satisfaction of infantile dependence was threatened. Marked lack of energy and courage was noted.' Asthmatics tend to have the same sort of personality, with the difference that they are usually 'less narcissistic . . . and much more vigorous and socially acceptable . . .'. Sufferers from coronary disease usually have a great need and respect for authority, are unremitting workers, who stick to one occupation and plan their career; they are compulsive (that is, feel bound to follow rules and rituals meticulously).[2] The types of disorders, however, which are found to be correlated with psychological factors seem to be much more numerous than those which yield to psychotherapeutic treatment, and even among the latter group the success of such treatment seems to vary from patient to patient.

The classification of certain disorders as 'psychosomatic' has been hotly attacked by some physicians who have successfully treated them by drugs, surgery or a special régime, and as hotly defended by those who have alleviated them by one form of psychotherapy or another. Suspicion has also been thrown upon it by metaphysicians, some of whom do not believe in Descartes' distinction in kind between body and mind, some of whom believe in it so strongly that they conceive of all interaction between the two as necessarily conscious and voluntary. The whole controversy is a good example of the dangers of forgetting that medicine is really a technique and not a science. It is regarded as scientific to classify disorders by symptom and by cause (for example, bacterial endocarditis), and this classification, coupled with the mind-

---

[1] By such workers as J. L. Halliday in Scotland and Flanders Dunbar in the U.S.A.

[2] 'Personality in Psychosomatic Disorders', E. F. Gildea, in *Psychosomatic Medicine* for September/October, 1949.

body dichotomy, leads to the creation of a false class—disorders with somatic symptoms and psychic causes. When physicians are not trying to be scientists or metaphysicians, however, they employ a much more practical classification of disorders, according to the method chosen for treating them. Patients in hospitals are separated into surgical, medical and psychiatric wards. This is a true technician's classification, and can be applied to the definition of psychosomatic disorders, which are really no more than bodily symptoms which some people treat successfully by the means used to treat mental symptoms. Just as some peptic ulcers are treated by surgery and some by diet, so asthma is sometimes treated by drugs and sometimes by psychotherapy; and metaphysics are as irrelevant in the latter case as in the former.[1]

Recommended Reading

PSYCHOSOCIAL MEDICINE, by J. L. Halliday. Heinemann, 1948.
EMOTIONS AND BODILY CHANGES, by Flanders Dunbar. Columbia University Press, 1946.

[1] I have argued this point of view at greater length in 'The Definition of Psychosomatic Disorder' in the *British Journal for the Philosophy of Science*, 1956.

INDEX OF NAMES

INDEX OF SUBJECTS